BRB

A Memoir About Coming
of Age in the Digital Age

LAUREN ELLMAN

Cover illustration by James Wight
and interior design by Euan Monaghan.

ISBN: 978-0-5788500-2-3

Ellie Jude, my entire life is dedicated to you.
You are my inspiration, my guru, my guiding light.
Thank you. Mommy loves you.

Chapter 1: Coming of Age in the Digital Age

MISSED CONNECTION: The year was 1998. I was a second-grade girl in jean short overalls and butterfly clips holding back my unruly bangs. You were Jonathan Taylor Thomas.

I am a member of what society refers to as the millennial generation. Please, please... hold your applause.

Yes, I am a proud product of the 1990s, raised on Nickelodeon slime, dial-up Internet and Red Dye No. 3. My room was wallpapered with glossy photos of boy bands and bubblegum pop stars. I wore the same pair of glittery black platform Sketcher sneakers every single day until they literally fell apart, because I desperately believed I was going to grow up to become Scary Spice. I once wrote a heartfelt letter to Zac Hanson and made my mom take a picture of me wearing an oversized Hanson t-shirt to send to him as fan mail. I fantasized about how he'd receive it, fall madly in love with me, and write back his marriage proposal. Maybe it got lost in the mail?

This is all to say, I had a very typical childhood.

The era of the 24-hour news cycle was just at its precipice, and people were glued to their television sets watching OJ Simpson's white Ford Bronco zipping down the highway in a live action police chase and reading articles in the newspaper about the mysterious murder of a child beauty queen. In order to keep up, the news needed to become more flashy and more sensationalized than ever before.

When I wasn't arguing with my friends over which Backstreet Boy was best (AJ, obviously), I was usually behind a screen. You see, I grew up with John Walsh of *America's Most Wanted* telling my parents I'd be abducted if I played outside. So, I went inside and played on the Internet, without much supervision, because our parents didn't really know what it was yet.

As early as elementary school, my friends and I had our own computers in our bedrooms, where we could surf the web and land anywhere we wanted. It was a whole new frontier and we, the millennials, were the first frontiersmen.

I was a precocious kid, the only daughter of two doting and overprotective parents. As their only child after multiple miscarriages, it makes total sense that they were terrified of something ever happening to me. And with the media constantly assuring them that something would, undoubtedly, happen to me, they taught me how to be terrified right along with them.

I was that kid at the first grade school carnival who kept asking for a new can of soda every time I left mine unattended, because I knew if I were to drink from that can again, it would definitely have roofies in it.

I was that kid who had her Halloween candy checked for razor blades.

I was that kid on the leash at Disney.

I was *that* kid.

Is it any surprise that I developed an unrelenting anxiety disorder?

I was raised to be fearful of my surroundings, and that fear bled into pretty much every other aspect of my life. As you'll see, my entire life has been underlined by this sense of fear and it always seemed justified. I was just being cautious or ambitious or smart. Unbeknownst to me and my parents, this fear manifested into an anxiety disorder.

//

One of my earliest memories is lying awake in my parents' bed, cradled between their two safe bodies, humming myself to sleep to drown out the thoughts racing through my head.

There was a period of about six months in fourth grade where I threw up every single night. All over my parents' bed. And bathroom. And feet.

I saw doctor after doctor who couldn't give us any reason why. I was told I might be allergic to certain foods. I should try not eating after a certain time.

I never mentioned that I was obsessively preoccupied with the idea of everyone I love dropping dead. Or how the thought of taking a standardized test brought on the adrenaline rush of a high-speed roller coaster. Or that sometimes I'd just feel this buzzy, scary feeling in my belly and not know how else to get rid of it.

Not even one of them ever even came close to suggesting the word *anxiety*. The word never came on our radar. And so it was brushed off as a lengthy stomach bug.

Even after years of spontaneous vomiting, tumultuous mood swings and migraines so severe I would fill a kitchen pot with ice water and submerge my head in it just to feel relief, I never once thought that I may be sick. I just went about my business, coming of age in the digital age.

//

I came online around middle school. The year was 2002, I had finally mastered Rainbow Run on Mario Kart, my AIM screen name was *sHoPaHoLiC1234* and if I ever accidentally sent a text from the brick of a cell phone my mom gave me for emergencies, I would have been grounded for eternity.

Around that time, everyone was building AOL Homepages. For those of you Gen Z-ers who aren't familiar, imagine spinning Word Art, low-quality glitter graphics and *lots* of Comic Sans. I spent hours a day chatting on AIM, crafting cryptic away messages with lyrics from Dashboard Confessional songs and getting angry every time someone called the house and kicked me off-line. I had a very active Live Journal account with lengthy posts all about the trials and tribulations of being an angsty eighth grader. I, of course, had a Myspace page where I learned how to code and rate my friends in batches of eight. And I got most of my sexual education from illegally downloaded and *very* explicit rap songs by Ludacris and his pals.

Then, when I was a sophomore in high school, Facebook happened. I was late to that game. Most people had one before me. It was just for college students at first, and I wasn't cool enough to know anyone with a college email to get myself an account. But then my friend set me up, and so began my torrid love affair with social media.

We were the first frontiersmen of the internet, and we had no idea what we were getting ourselves into. No one really did. Not even the people creating it. But technology accelerates at such an exponential rate, there is no way we could have braced ourselves for the upheaval social media was about to wreck on our culture.

We used to have the vague, general concept of "society" telling us what was true and who we should be and what we should think. Now, society has a megaphone named social media and it is infiltrating every aspect of our waking lives.

There is a clear intersection where mental health and social media overlap. And I believe it's imperative that we explore that intersection in order to better guard ourselves and our mental health from the negative side effects of that overlap. Getting to know ourselves, our true selves, before society and social media told us who to be, is the very first step in safeguarding our mental health. The stronger our understanding of ourselves, the better equipped we become to coexist with these new technologies. The more we tune into our own voices, the less we believe the voices that are screaming at us from the millions of pieces of online content we consume every day.

The problem is that the technology is so advanced and has been specifically designed to know us better than we know ourselves. At least, that's the promise that they make when selling their product. Think about it. Do you pay to use Facebook? Instagram? Twitter? No. Then who pays? Advertising companies. And what are they paying for? Our attention. We are the product. Rather, the promise that our behavior can be manipulated and changed is the product. And social media companies can offer that promise with almost absolute certainty based on their predictions. And prediction certainty needs lots and lots of data.

We know this. We know they are tracking what we engage with and when and for how long. But do we fully understand what the tracking affords them? Imagine if we could buy back our own data and see what they know about us. Learn what triggers us; what makes us tick.

How can we expect to trust our own internal nudges, those alarms that go off when something doesn't feel true, when there are scientists and artificial intelligence programs collecting data to learn how to nudge us harder, better and faster? They nudge us with notifications and curated feeds and echo chambers that reaffirm the worldview they've manufactured for us. How can we stand a chance against that?

Well, I believe we can. I believe we must. Social media and tech companies are the ultimate gaslighters. They've been feeding us misinformation and programming us to doubt ourselves for years. It's gotten to the point where we never know what's really true. But it is possible to survive and overcome the torment of a gaslighter.

Now, before I crack open and dig into my particularly hellish and toxic relationship with social media, let's get back to that little girl in second grade for a moment, the one in the jean overalls with glittery metal butterflies atop her frizzy helmet of hair. I think she has something to teach us.

Chapter 2: Who Are You, Really?

I've always been really good at not giving a fuck about what people thought about me. I consider it my superpower. I mean, middle school was a three-year-long dumpster fire, and I certainly had my share of self-conscious moments. But for the most part, I've been able to beat to my own drum and not care if anyone else enjoyed the music.

This may have had to do with my parents believing the literal sun shined out of my ass. Or because I'm one of the lucky, entitled few born into the millennial generation, so I intrinsically think I'm the best at everything because I always got a trophy. But I like to think it's just something I was born with.

I never really understood what was *cool* by my peers' standards, insisting instead on defining the word for myself. I was also very lucky in that my parents always encouraged me to stay true to myself. They certainly weren't paying attention to the trends, so I never was.

That's why in second grade, when picture day rolled around and every other girl was choosing which Limited Too graphic tee to wear and having their moms weave intricate French braids into their hair, I chose to gather up my bangs and string them into a single strand of rainbow beads in the middle of my forehead. I completed my picture day ensemble with a pink-and-white-striped shirt with Tweety Bird in the center, worn under a pair of jean overalls and a beaded choker necklace I had made by hand. It's why I always chose Lance as my favorite member of NSYNC, because no one else seemed to. It's why I played with dolls well into middle school. It's why that day at summer camp, when all the popular girls were making the shape of an L on their foreheads and laughing at me, I was able to shrug it off.

My clothes were always a little different, my hair always a little messier, my laugh always a little louder and more boisterous. But, I *enjoyed* being myself. I was a silly, sarcastic smart-ass with a heart of gold. And somewhere, deep beneath the layers of wear and tear and multiple identity crises over the last thirty years, that little smart-ass is still in there, keeping that fire in my belly alive. She's there with a quick-witted comeback whenever I need one. She's there to insist that I can do whatever I want in this life. She's there to remind me that there's good in everyone.

What I'm realizing now, as a semi-functional adult, is that it is my duty, my responsibility, to keep in touch with her. Trust her. Let her lead.

Sure, I've given in to peer pressure more than once. Getting drunk at the big party, pretending to laugh at the frat boy's lame jokes, waking up hungover and regretful the next morning. Spending money I didn't have on clothes I didn't like. Ditching my real friends to try hanging with the "popular" kids. But, for the most part, I'm proud to say I've stayed true to myself. But the only way to do that is by listening to that little nudge of intuition inside that alerts me when something doesn't feel true. And trusting that what may be true for others doesn't have to be true for me.

It takes a lot of work and dedication to stay in touch with it, but over the years I've decided it's my best shot to safeguard my mental health from the incessant noise that's rushing at me from every direction.

That little nudge of intuition I'm talking about is our true self. Our inner child. Our truth. We need to search within and find the line between who we are and who we've learned to be. And the first step in that journey is remembering who we used to be before everyone was watching.

//

In second grade, there was a girl with a learning disability in our class. Her name was Raquel. She was the first person with a learning disability that I had ever met. While other kids chose to disregard her as "weird" or "broken," I took a seat next to her and became her friend.

One day, while she was in the bathroom, a boy opened the door on her. The bathroom was inside the classroom, so the entire class saw this happen. I'm not sure if he didn't know someone was in there or if he was just being a little asshole, but nevertheless the entire class watched as Raquel hurriedly pulled her pants up, shrieking, with toilet paper hanging out of her waistband. They all snickered under their breaths, mocking her for putting toilet paper down on the seat (I never understood why that was something to mock; I still do that to this day. Can't squat, won't squat). Her face went bright red and she ran out of the room sobbing.

While our teacher tried and failed to quiet the class down, I chased after her.

I don't remember what I said. I just remember hugging her. I remember feeling her brown frizzy hair beneath my hands as I rubbed her back. I remember feeling her tears on my shoulder. I don't think I had ever felt someone else's tears before. I want to believe that something I did or something I said helped her understand that she didn't need to give a fuck about what those kids thought. She was so much smarter and braver and better than them. I want to believe I helped her see that in that moment.

I'm not sure what happened to Raquel. I don't think she continued at our school after that year. But I'll never forget her.

Over the years, I continued to do the same for anyone and everyone I felt was being mistreated. From the "bad" kid who always got in trouble with the teacher to the quiet girl who everyone thought was "crazy" because she was shy and didn't know English very well to the "scary" girl who thought she was a witch. I always sidled up next to them and became their friend. Everyone needs a champion. Everyone needs someone in their corner.

The girl who thought she was a witch was named Katie. Everyone else wrote her off as "weird" or "scary," which always made me want to befriend her more.

In fourth grade we had a class recital one evening after school. All the kids were gathered in a random classroom waiting to go on stage. It was so exciting to be in school at nighttime, we were all buzzing about, taking it all in. Then I noticed Katie in the corner, sitting at a desk with her head rested upon her arms. It looked like she was crying. Everyone else was screaming and laughing around her, as if she wasn't even there. But all I could see was her thin frame, slumped over in small, steady sobs. It was louder than all the energetic fourth graders showing off their "nighttime personas."

I went to her.

I sat down in the empty seat next to hers and asked, "Are you okay?"

She was visibly startled. She picked up her head and her eyes were red, her cheeks wet with tears. She looked at me and shook her head. Her eyes looked around at nothing in particular, trying to find words.

"My dog died today," she said, her mouth saying something her heart obviously didn't want to believe.

My heart broke for her. My dog, Rex, had died that year as well. I remembered how hard it was. The pain I felt. The tears I cried. I instantly empathized with Katie. I felt her pain. My compassion for her was visceral.

I put my arm around her as she bowed her head again, tears dropping one by one down onto the desk. We just sat there together for a minute, my presence offering her as much comfort as it could.

"I don't want to do this stupid recital," she spit out.

I looked her right in the eye and nodded once, as if to say, "I'm on it."

I went up to whatever adult was in the room and told them the situation. I said someone should get Katie's dad because she can't do the recital.

He found her sitting at that same desk, with me silently alongside her. She ran into his arms and burst into heavier sobs, the ones she was holding back. He thanked me for being there for her. And then they were gone.

Moments just like this have sprung up time and again throughout my life. And my natural reaction has always been the same. *Go to them.* My inner-child is still in there, pulling me toward other people, reminding me to find that common thread that links us all together.

Social media has tried to shut that little girl up, has tested her compassion and has jaded her worldview. From dreadful news stories to unrealistic beauty ideals to the inevitable notification that my ex had moved on without me, that confident, hopeful little girl has been knocked down. But, if I sink down deep enough, to that spot where all the noise slows to a low hum, I can get back in touch with her. And she's always there, patiently waiting for my return with a smile on her face and her arms open wide, her brilliant eyes saying, *welcome home.*

//

At some point, we all attach ourselves to this idea of who we are. We call it our identity. We drape ourselves with layers of labels and styles and likes and dislikes. *I'm outdoorsy, I'm a vegan, I'm an influencer, I'm a sports fanatic, I'm an academic, I'm a man's man, I'm a feminist, I'm a mom, I'm a boss.*

I'm… *full of shit.*

Don't get me wrong. I totally get subscribing to things that bring you joy and make you feel good or purposeful or proud. But I can't get behind gleaning our entire identity from those things. They're all external and ever-evolving. The only thing you are and will always be is you. Everything else is just decoration.

Maybe we all eventually fall into this trap as a mechanism to cope with our need to fit into society. Like we need to pick a tribe to join. We need to fit in. But I'm afraid we're losing who we really are at our core in the process.

It's as if we all have this version of ourselves that we've made up, like a character in a story. And we attach attributes to that character. A sense of style. Hobbies. A favorite drink. A political affiliation. A taste in music. We believe that's our identity, who we are. But it's fabricated. Made up. Not real.

Worse, parts of it have been covertly programmed into us by social media. These big tech companies and their advertising customers make billions of dollars exploiting the vulnerability of human psychology. They pay big money to learn where to find us and how to get in front of us, covertly infiltrating our News Feeds without us even realizing. They aren't just given access to our data, they are given access to the algorithm that best targets us. They create campaigns to manufacture a specific echo chamber that we then exist within online, learning how to dress, speak, think, and behave, all to benefit their own bottom line.

Some consequences of that business model are mild. For example, a fast fashion company pays to show up in front of busy moms and attempts to convince us that their latest line of athleisure is what we *need*. *Look at all of these other busy moms drinking their coffee and killing it in these new leggings.* Since we've subscribed to this idea that we are a member of the #busymom squad, we may spend money we don't have on leggings we don't need simply to quench that subconscious thirst to fit in. I'm a busy mom; busy moms wear these leggings. Therefore, I need these leggings.

Did you know that the polyester, nylon, spandex, and acrylic in those leggings are all synthetic fibers derived from petroleum? They make up about sixty-five percent of our clothes and are favored by manufacturers because they provide a cheap and fast alternative to natural fibers. Therefore, both that fast fashion company and oil companies have a mutual interest in promoting those leggings to us, via the algorithm that we're guided into online— and they're willing to pay big bucks to do so.

And, if an oil company can make billions ruining the earth and depleting resources, it isn't a stretch to imagine that same corporation creating a viral campaign via social media to easily convince people global warming is a hoax. When corporations have the power to convince citizens that science isn't real in order to benefit their own bottom line, we're in trouble.

With social media, this happens every day and has been happening for a while. Access to the algorithm is afforded to the highest bidder, and we're all complicit. We willingly participate because we're addicts. Of course we are. We don't stand a chance. They designed this technology to behave like the most seductive and addictive drug on the market. We're users. And they prey on our vulnerability. Rather than using it as a tool to connect and learn, we use it for dopamine hits and confirmation that we're well-liked and fitting in.

But, I sense the tides turning. I see user after user sobering up, myself included. We are ready and willing to drop out of the matrix and get back in touch with our true selves. The sooner we all do that, the sooner we can come back and use these technologies as tools instead of as drugs. But we first need to remember who we were before they told us who to be.

I believe, at our core, we all have one single unchanging essence. It doesn't morph or transition as we do throughout life. It's who we were as a little kid when no one was watching. Full of wonder and innocence, before we were corrupted by the world. We've all been that little kid. Some of us lose it sooner than others, but if we try hard enough I bet we can all think back and remember how it felt. And I think it's necessary that we tap into that core, that essence of who we really are, before we become so disassociated with reality that we can't make our way back.

//

When I was four years old, my mom surprised me with a dollhouse. I woke up on the third night of Hanukkah to a pink and blue Fisher-Price dollhouse waiting for me in my bedroom. Completely furnished, with little people strewn about just waiting for me to create entire lives for them. I spent what feels like my entire childhood tucked behind that dollhouse, weaving intricate narratives for each character and playing God with their plastic little lives.

The little plastic children had a miniature dollhouse, a replica of the one they lived in. And I remember positioning the blonde brother and sister to sit and play with their dollhouse and coming upon my very first existential thought.

*Maybe they're coming up with little lives for their dolls in their house just like I'm coming up with little lives for them. And if **that's** true, maybe I'm just a doll in someone else's bigger dollhouse and they're playing with **me**.*

Ever since I can remember, I've had this sneaking suspicion that we aren't as in control as we think we are. We can't control time. We can't control events. And we especially can't control other people. Their bigger person with their bigger dollhouse is in charge of that.

No, the only thing that we can control, the only thing that is ours and ours alone, is our sense of self. Who we are. We get to control that. We get to decide who we show up as in this world.

But the work lies in piecing together who we are and why. What has been inherited, learned, or forced onto us. What parts have we outgrown, what parts are we proud of, what parts have we forgotten about.

I don't think I was born anxious. I think it's something I inherited. But for a long time, I thought of it as an intrinsic part of who I am. I *am* anxious. I am a perfectionist. I avoid confrontation. I need order.

I assigned these labels to myself, and it's only now, as I'm starting to take responsibility for my recovery, that I'm poking holes in all of those "truths" I have so fervently believed for years.

I'm not anxious; I just fear uncertainty. I'm not a perfectionist; I'm just afraid of failure. I don't avoid confrontation; I just don't speak up for myself. I don't need order; I just place importance on it in a veiled attempt to assume control.

I am merely a product of my upbringing. Salacious news stories coupled with doting, protective parents, left me primed for an anxiety disorder. Understanding that has helped me better understand myself. I am not my anxiety. Rather, my anxiety is a tenant in my mind. A tenant among many other qualities that signed their lease long before I understood I was their landlord.

This understanding has helped me piece together other parts of my personality. Whether it was the characters that have come in and out of my life over the last 30 years, the environment in which I was raised or simply the generation I was born into, I am a sum of these parts.

A big part of my identity lives in memories I've forgotten, moments from what feels like another lifetime. In taking the time to dive inward and unpack that, I've been able to examine who I truly am and see that a lot of my personality comes from my family. Parts of my personality that I always thought were inherently "me," upon reflection, are clearly inherited.

For example, when I am being louder than necessary, that's my mother's father, my Papa Hector. When I go into hermit mode and retreat into my shell with fear and worry, that's his wife, my Mimi. When I'm getting pissy and bitter, that's my father's mother, Nanny. And when I get heated, like red-in-the-face angry, that's my Papa

Jack. If we look long enough, with open eyes, we can trace so many parts of ourselves back to who we've come from and how we were brought up.

Aside from who raised me, I know a lot of "truths" I believe about myself come from past experiences that informed my self-perception. Being told by an ex-boyfriend that I'm always afraid of everything, for example, planted a seed that eventually grew roots inside my psyche and I convinced myself it was true. On the flip side, being told by my fifth-grade teacher that I'm a talented writer led me to pursue that talent, practice it, and improve upon it. So many reflections of myself from other people's perspectives have told me who I am, and it's only now as I take my thirtieth trip around the sun that I'm learning I need to unpack those boxes and sift through what's my truth and what's theirs.

Some of my inner world has been inherited, some has been reflected back at me and some, still, has been programmed into me by the media. What was once child stars in glossy magazine spreads telling me what clothes to wear and how to talk to boys, is now social media influencers and viral marketing campaigns telling me how to keep my house, raise my kids, what to read, where to shop, who to like, what to drink. The list is endless.

When you pay close enough attention, it's easy to connect the dots and see how much of what we consider our personal identity is tied back to what we see in our News Feeds. For example, my corner of the internet, where the millennial #busymoms hang out, has taught me that wine and coffee are necessary fuels for motherhood, minimalism with three kids is totally possible and leggings are pants. Aside from the leggings-being-pants part, which I wholeheartedly support, those other things just aren't true for me. I feel awful when I drink alcohol or coffee, and trying to make my house look like Marie Kondo lives here is unrealistic. It took me unplugging for a minute to realize that those things don't need to be true *for me* for me to still "fit in" with other moms.

My newsfeed has also taught me a lot of positive truths, though. Like stretch marks are normal, other moms cry in the closet, and cereal can be dinner. It just took becoming a bit more mindful about who I was following and what type of content I was consuming for me to create a safe space for myself online, one that's authentic and feels good to participate in. I'm no longer *trying* to fit in. I'm simply showing up and finding my people along the way. These days, I'm connecting with them, learning from them, and feeling a lot less alone.

What's important to remember is that social media's effort to catch us and sell us something while we're scrolling is never going to cease. As long as advertisers are trying to make money and are given access to our algorithms, we will have to do our part to be a step ahead of them.

Scary news stories will always heighten my anxiety and picture-perfect #instamoms will always make me feel like I'm doing something wrong. Therefore, it's my job to be a conscious consumer of content and a vigilant gate keeper of what I allow in. I must pay attention to what truths I'm collecting and, every so often, call upon my old friend Marie Kondo and do some KonMari of the mind: *This truth no longer sparks joy, therefore I shall thank it and let it go.*

Along with the specific cocktail of media tactics, family members and life experiences that influence who we are, I still believe a large part of who we are is born with us. Each of us will always have that spark of essence, that flickering light that we were born with, swirling around in our core. That innocent, curious little kid. I like to think that's our intuition, the urgency in our gut when we know something is off and the voice in our head that says something amazing is about to happen.

In today's societal landscape of filters and hashtags and fake news and reality stars, I fear we're at risk of losing that spark forever. We spend so much time pretending to be who we think we're supposed to be, who we think we *want* to be, that we're losing touch with who we truly are.

We're disregarding the most beautiful parts of ourselves. The fallible, vulnerable, human parts of ourselves. Those parts don't make it online and, sadly, online is where we are all the time now.

We used to leave away messages that said BRB, ("be right back.") We don't say that anymore. We live here now.

We need to make it our life's work to care about ourselves and get to know ourselves, in each new season of life. And this self-care

doesn't live in the picture you post of your feet in the bathtub followed by #selfcare. It's not in the 280 characters you tweet about
your revelatory ayahuasca journey. And it certainly isn't drinking
celery juice every morning because you saw some girl on Instagram
doing it.

No.

Self-care is the daily dedication to the self. We can't show up
online until we commit to showing up for ourselves in person. We
can't let algorithms know us better than we know ourselves. It's
our responsibility to take care of ourselves and nurture that spark
of essence inside, so that we can better take care of those around
us. What a world we could live in if we all got our heads out of our
proverbial asses, put our phones down, and started seeing each other
for what we really are. Innocent, curious little kids.

Chapter 3: Mi Gente

"Can we just agree...there is no Christmas...in this house?," my husband says to me, stretching out the pauses between his words for emphasis.

This past weekend, my stepson committed an act of sacrilege when he asked my mother if he could take a toy from her house. Of course, being a doting grandmother who lives to spoil her grandchildren, she said yes. The thing about this toy is that it was an elf. Not just any elf. But a Christmas elf. And as my husband so kindly likes to remind me, "We don't do Christmas at our house."

"You want me to take the toy away from him because it's dressed in red and green," I state, more than ask.

"We don't celebrate Christmas here," he repeats.

"It's not like he's skipping around a tree with it singing Jingle Bells. It's a toy, he likes it. Does it really bother you that much that it's red and green?"

"You know what I mean. It's a Christmas thing. We don't do Christmas here. We don't celebrate that. We're Jewish. We celebrate Hanukkah."

I would have been able to drop this argument if we were just two adults in a disagreement. However, our children were involved. They hear him say things like this. And I refuse to raise children who are uneducated about or —worse—intolerant of other cultures, beliefs, and values. But more than that, I'm stubborn beyond all reason. So, of course, I press on.

"What if our neighbors were telling their kids they can't play with dreidels because they don't do that in their house? That's something the Jews do. We aren't Jews. We do Christmas here. Let them keep the dreidels in their homes."

"I don't want to talk about this anymore. You're just becoming argumentative."

You're damn right I was being argumentative. It's what I do best, after all. But what do you expect a child's logical conclusion to be after hearing this sort of rhetoric? You're teaching them that there's an Us and a Them. We do things our way; they do things another way. We're separate.

What happens when they learn that Christmas is celebrated as Jesus' birthday, and that some people believe that Jesus is their savior, pray to him, and base their values around his teachings. Why *wouldn't* they reject those people as "others?" *Don't bring your Christmas or your Jesus or your bible to our house. We don't "do" that here.*

Are you kidding me?

This coming from the man who repeatedly stands on his soap box preaching that his country is the earth and his religion is doing good. That we're all brothers and sisters and there are no boundaries between us. How can you honestly claim to believe that while claiming that we can't have a red and green elf toy in the house because, *we don't do that here?*"

Obviously, this is about *so* much more than a stupid little elf toy.

"Judaism is about the home, Lauren," says my husband, the atheist who brags about how he denounced Judaism once he realized that it was "just a brainwashing mechanism to indoctrinate people into following orders."

"We aren't any less Jewish if we celebrate and accept other cultures and religions."

"We're Jewish. We need to maintain our heritage. We need to keep our history alive through the children and how we run our home."

My eyebrows bunch together, clearly showing I'm not about to let this go.

"Can we just agree that there's no Christmas in this house?"

"No."

He rolls his eyes, convinced I'm just trying to win an argument. Convinced I'm just being stubborn. Convinced I'm faking the rage behind my words.

I continue, frustratedly looking for the right words and coming up short. "No, because that's small-minded. You're full of shit. And I refuse to raise my kids that way."

I'm not sure of his reaction, because it happened on the opposite side of the door I slammed and walked out of.

//

It's the year 2000. I'm ten years old, in the throes of fifth grade, and finally off for winter break.

"Feliz Navidad, prospero año y Felicidaaaad," Jose Feliciano sings to me from the boombox perched atop our dining room table.

I'm home with my mom, who is hunkered down in her own makeshift Christmas workshop. Silver bells litter the floor, gobs of dried hot glue gather at the edges of the table, tinsel and pine needles stick to the bottom of my dirty bare feet. She is creating Christmas wreaths to give to our friends and family. I help by picking out what to glue, where.

"Mommy, what about this little elf?," I call from the couch as I watch her. I pull out a tiny, plastic figurine from between the cushions. I hold out the Christmas elf, who has red and green stripes across his pointy hat.

"Perfecto!" She takes the gun against his back and lets the hot glue spread, burning the tips of her fingers just a bit.

"I wanna wish you a Merry Christmas, from the bottom of my heart," I sing along with Jose, mimicking his heavy Cuban accent, as I prance around my crafting mother.

Christmastime. I look forward to it every year. Sure, the time off from school is great. And the presents don't hurt. But the reason I look forward to Christmas so much is because of how happy my mom becomes. She's smiling, singing, dancing, glowing. I get to spend lots of time with her, decorating the house and wrapping presents and shopping for gifts.

As a kid, my mom worked a lot. After I started elementary school, she started her own business with her business partner Carlos. She was usually stressed, rushing out of the house, taking late night phone calls, chain-smoking behind my back. I didn't always get to spend time with her. I never noticed back then, to be honest. It was just normal. She spent a lot of time with Carlos, while I stayed home with my dad. He and I would eat dinner in front of the TV while we battled each other in Jeopardy and Wheel of Fortune. My mom just worked a lot.

Except for Christmas. Christmas was her favorite time of year, and it became mine as well. She'd be home a lot more, decorating, shopping, cooking, and planning. And I got to do it all with her.

Over time, less and less of the decorations would make it back to the garage until one year she just left them all up. Including the tree. At our house, it was always Christmas. And that's something I secretly loved, as bizarre as it may have been to explain a Christmas tree to my friends in the middle of July. I loved it because it reminded me of happier times.

//

For context, I am a second-generation Cuban American Jew who grew up in the suburbs of Miami. Spanish was my first language. But if you met me today, you wouldn't peg me for a Cuban. My blonde hair, blue eyes, and vegetarian diet don't really scream *Oye, mi gente!* (Hey, my people!) I don't even drink coffee anymore (gasp!). But growing up, being Cuban was an integral part of my identity.

I spent so much time at my grandparents' house that even to this day it serves as the backdrop to every dream I have. The brown shaggy carpet. The blue tins of shortbread cookies scattered about the house, some with cookies, others with sewing needles or cotton balls or coupons. The *telenovelas* screaming in rapid-fire Spanish on the TV set, as my grandfather rocked back and forth in his beige leather recliner. The house always smelled like *cafecito*. No matter what time of day, you'd walk in and be greeted with the fierce aroma of Cuban coffee and sugar brewing from a tiny, silver kettle sitting at the very edge of fiery orange coils on the stovetop. Every party had the same soundtrack: ceramic dominos being clacked around on plastic tables, Celia Cruz's deep vibrato assuring us that life was, indeed, a carnival, and loud, loud, **loud** voices, drunk on rum coming from lungs filled with cigar smoke.

This is the lifeblood that runs through my veins. This is a significant part of the fabric that makes me who I am. And yet, I don't get to really share it with my family now. That wonderful house with the brown shag carpet has long been sold. Those loud, loud voices of *tios* and *vecinos* and *sobrinos* are all gone. That beige leather recliner no longer rocks back and forth.

//

My *abuelo*, Papa Hector, was the most eccentric character you'd ever know. Born in Cuba, he left with his family in 1959 as Fidel Castro came to power. Leaving with nothing, he brought his wife, my Mimi, my mother and her younger brother first to Madrid, then to New York City, and finally settled everyone down in Miami, where a good chunk of Cuban political refugees put down roots.

Papa Hector was loud. Louder than you're thinking. Loud like you could hear him long before you could see him. He had jet black hair that was always wet and greased back and to the side with a comb. He was a thin man with a pot belly, his belly button jutting out the front, and thin, almost feminine legs. Hairless. He'd show them off in teeny, tiny metallic-colored speedos and even g-strings when he'd go to the beach. He'd frequent his fair share of nudist beaches across Europe on vacation. He also purchased an apartment on Miami Beach with a balcony overlooking the shore, just so he could sit perched atop it and use his binoculars to peep on the topless sunbathers.

This was my grandfather. The loud, energetic, ridiculous, loving, intelligent, preposterous nudist. He was the love of my life. My best friend. My firmest genetic link to what I believe I am made of.

//

I was a stubborn brat when I was a teenager. Some would argue not much has changed.

It was an exceptionally warm Miami day, in July 2005. I had just turned fifteen and was dating some kid I couldn't get enough of.

That night, he was coming over to watch a movie. I was eager to get home from my job as a summer camp counselor to get ready.

"We need to stop at your *abuelo's* before we go home," my mom said as she turned off 8th Street and toward their house.

"Oh my god, mom! Do we have to? I just want to get home." The thought of how bratty I must've sounded makes me cringe.

"Just for a minute, then we'll go home."

"Ugh. Fine. But I'm not getting down." I crossed my arms against my chest in protest.

"*Por favor* Lauren, just say hi to them."

"No, I don't feel good. I'll just see them tomorrow."

She rolled her eyes, dropped the argument, and pulled into their driveway. I stayed in the car.

That night, as I was groping my new boyfriend on the couch, not watching a movie, my mom ran into the room.

She was frantic. A look on her face unlike one I'd ever seen.

"I'm going to Mimi and Papa's. My dad just had a stroke."

Her dad. My grandfather. My Papa. The love of my life. The man who used to tell my mom to "let me make memories" whenever she didn't let me do something fun. The man who would strut around Miami Beach in a bright yellow g-string, binoculars strung around his chest to get a better view of the topless ladies. The man who would let me sit on his lap and mess up his perfectly greased black hair. The man whose voice was so loud, I can still feel it booming in my chest. The man who gave me the *cojones* to stand up for myself, to make myself heard, to be as loud and obnoxious as I need to be in order to get what I want. Her dad. My grandfather. My Papa.

He had a stroke that night. He didn't survive. And I stayed in the car.

//

That day is forever seared into my memory. The regret of not getting out of that car that afternoon is something I still can't shake, fifteen years later.

I cried so hard, I can still feel those sobs ripping through me. I begged God through gut-wrenching sobs on my bathroom floor to bring my grandfather back, to give me one more chance. If He could please give me just one more chance, I'd do it right. I would get out of the car. I would give him one last hug.

But I'd never really *spoken* to God, never a conversation. It was always me pleading with him for answers. I never formed a friendship with him (her/it/them); never gave him the chance to speak back. Not until that night in the desert.

We arrived at the Negev Desert in southern Israel late at night. I was there on my Birthright trip, a free opportunity for every Jewish person to visit Israel. It is seen as our "birthright" to visit the homeland because, in the Jewish culture, it is essential that we know where we come from. It is a chance to learn about our roots and experience our heritage. Friends who took their trip before me told me it would change my life. I would come back a new person with a new insight and sense of connection to my heritage. Twenty-year-old me didn't really understand. I expected Israel to just be sand and camels.

That night, our trip leader Gedalia, an armed Israeli soldier, led our group into the desert. He prefaced the hike with a quick request.

"It is going to be very dark out there," he began. His Israeli accent made the English words sound more important, as if they demanded our attention.

"Please do not bring any flashlights," he continued. "You might stumble on a rock or two, but your eyes will get accustomed to the darkness." All twenty-four of us looked around at each other and then out into the black wall of night awaiting us. The only light for miles was a single street lamp standing above us, illuminating our desert campsite.

"And one more thing," he said, a bit louder to regain our attention. He paused for a second to make sure all of our eyes were on him. "You must not speak until we are back at the campsite. Understood?"

"Understood," we answered in a collective, anxious whisper.

And so began our hike into the total darkness.

There was no light in the desert but the moon shining overhead. Prickly branches and jagged rocks surprised my feet as I stumbled over them. My heart began to race as I peered at the black sheet of night that lay ahead of me. I picked up my head for a moment to look around, curious to see if everyone else felt as nervous as I did. But I couldn't see a single other person, only shadowy figures stumbling around like me as they tried to follow the path. Finally, after what felt like hours, our hike came to a halt. Gedalia's voice was the only one to break the silence.

"Welcome to the Negev Desert," he said. "Where you are standing now, Moses stood."

I felt that rush through me. I looked down at my feet, amazed.

"According to the Torah, he used to come out here and speak to God."

I felt a twinge of cynicism. I never considered my relationship with God to be very serious. God, to me, was like a long-distance pen pal. I made an effort to keep in touch, but I didn't really know him and I could never see him. And I didn't really count on him for much. I believed that I was in control. I made things happen. A simple cause and effect philosophy. I was too stubborn to get out of the car to see Papa; therefore I never got to say goodbye. I was to blame for my misfortunes. I was the center of my own universe. But as I stood there, staring at the millions of shining stars sprinkled over the black sky, I suddenly felt very small.

Gedalia asked us each to find a spot alone in the desert to sit and reflect. I sat down on a small rock and felt it beneath me, supporting me. It was just big enough to fit my entire bottom, which wasn't very big at all, and it was covered in sand. But it was cool to the touch, so cool I could feel goose bumps all over my legs.

The landscape around me seemed not of this world. The desert spanned farther than I could imagine. Shadows of small, bristly trees sprouted up every few yards or so, the wind briefly stirring and sending sand dancing through the air and then into my eyes. But only for a second. Then the wind was gone and the silence set in. The silence is what captivated me most. Not a single sound could be heard. I noticed I was holding my breath in fear of disturbing it. The only thing I could hear were the thoughts in my head. And in the silent desert, they sounded so clear. I could finally *listen* to them.

I took a deep breath and shut my eyes. As I blinked them back open, I could see it. The universe. The whole entire universe sprawling out in front of me in all its infinite glory.

In the distance, I could see the faint silhouette of the mountains. I couldn't see a single other person through the darkness. It was just me and the desert and the universe. And I felt very small. Every worry I had ever had suddenly seemed to shrink into dust. I couldn't even remember the last thing I worried about. Was it if my boyfriend had called me? Or was it if I should study Hebrew when I got back home? It all seemed so insignificant when I was staring at the big picture. I let my eyes pan over the sky, dumbfounded. Once I took it all in, I closed my eyes once more, and let it swallow me whole.

That was the moment I realized what God is. God is the infinite, vast, all-encompassing universe that swirls around us and within us. Not to be touched or seen or understood. Just trusted. However you name that universe, whatever pronoun you give it, it doesn't matter. That's not the part that matters. What matters is connecting to it. Connecting to that source, that energy that has never been created or destroyed. It lives in infinity, breathing in and out of every single one of us, forever. That's **my** God.

My eyes were closed and my breath was deep. The breeze swirled around me, wrapping me in a blanket. It's as if someone was embracing me, rocking me back and forth, letting me know I'm taken care of. I felt Papa there in the desert beside me. I felt him kiss my forehead and rub my shoulders. He told me he'll be watching over me. He's been watching over me. My chest felt like I had just swallowed the sun. I didn't want to open my eyes in fear of losing him again. Then a gust of wind danced over my skin, giving my spine a quick shiver, and he was gone. I was alone again in the desert. I opened my eyes and looked at the sky. Millions of stars stared back at me. And then I tried to speak to God.

Hello, I said in my head, my eyes begging the stars to hear me. *I'm not very good at this but I just want to know if you're out there. I* waited a moment and suddenly felt another cool desert breeze whisk over my bare shoulders. An answer.

I don't really have anything to ask of you tonight. I don't have much to say at all, really. I was kind of hoping you might have something to say to me. I sat entirely still perched atop my rock, waiting, listening. The absolute desert silence let me listen. In the stillness, I felt a tidal wave of emotion consume me. It all rushed through me so fast I couldn't slow down to feel it. It rocked me awake from my meditation, throwing my eyes wide open. Suddenly, my bones felt stronger, my back sat straighter. I could hear.

God answered me. He showed me how expansive the universe is and how small and inconsequential my problems are in relation. He helped me see that I have the courage to give up control and really trust the universe. That I am the universe. We are all little pieces of the universe—little pieces of God that make up the whole. And as I relinquished my control to the many stars above, I never felt more powerful. And so I pleaded with God once again. I begged for the strength to hang onto this feeling. I prayed to keep it forever. I could already tell that it was fleeting, slipping through my desperate fingers as easily as the desert sand I was sitting upon. It would take me many years, possibly a lifetime, to ever really grab hold of that feeling and own it.

But as I sat there, tasting communion for the first time, I felt a smile sneak across my face. My mind was still, my heart was happy. I was sitting on a rock in the middle of the desert without a care in the world. I was completely alone. I sat on my rock as a new person, with a new insight and a new sense of connection.

//

I've always felt like all Jews are my family. I understood the genetic link. I've experienced the phenomenon of Jewish geography. I know how inherently connected we all are.

But sitting in the Negev, where Moses once stood, feeling the centuries of history that **my** people have lived, I really felt Jewish for the first time.

Growing up, my Jewish life was pretty peripheral. My family sat around a table every Passover and read the same stories and sang the same songs. We dipped the parsley in the salt water and I ran around feverishly looking for the *afikomen* while my older cousins snuck sips of *manischewitz* from the bottle. But we never really prayed or made an effort to connect to the Jewish story or spoke to God.

My father and his siblings had a much more stringent American-Jewish experience. My grandparents were devout Ashkenazi Jews of Russian and Austrian descent. My father and my aunts would spend every Saturday morning walking miles to the temple, and my dad spent most Sundays getting kicked out of bar mitzvah school by his unamused rabbi. My father's father, my Papa Jack, was very connected to Judaism. But for some reason, I never really was. It wasn't until going to Israel that I really began to identify with that part of my story. And it gave me the chance to find a very significant context to what "religion" means to me.

//

Being Jewish is something I am. It's my blood, my history, my story. But it's not my whole story. I wouldn't even say it's most of my story. Being Jewish is something I identify with. But being Cuban is something I feel in my bones.

It seems like in agreeing to run a Jewish household per my husband's request, I have inadvertently given up my right to include my children in my own heritage, my own story. And maybe I got so worked up over that stupid little elf, not because I'm afraid he's turning our kids into close-minded Christmas-haters, but because he's denying me the chance to share an enormous part of myself with my children. A part I didn't realize I missed so much until suddenly it was being taken away.

I've abandoned all the customs and traditions I grew up with as a child. The loud Noche Buena dinners. Jose Felicianos' rendition of "Feliz Navidad" blasting while Papa Hector pours more rum into the egg nog. Jingling bells. Clinking glasses. The smell of lechon and rice and beans. Men screaming over dominos. My grandfather's classic clip-on Christmas tie that lit up, illuminating his happy drunk face. Chaotic. And aromatic. And warm. And mine.

This is the fabric I wrap around my identity. The threads I pull together when I dip into moments of nostalgia. The place I revert back to when I feel homesick, for a time more than a place. A time

I miss. A time I desperately cling to. A time I wish more than anything I could invite my kids and my husband to be a part of.

But I can't.

I would give anything for the chance to take them to my grandparents' house for a typical Noche Buena dinner. For them to meet my wild grandfather and sit on his lap while he's dressed up as a drunk Santa Claus. To feel the warmth and the love. I'd love for them to see me as a little girl, sitting with my grandmother on her blue silk bed sheets while she taught me how to wrap presents. And her delicate handwriting as she addressed a personal label on each one: "From Santa Deju." They always had the biggest tree and it was littered with gifts underneath. Sometimes I'd play with their manger scene and my Barbies would pretend Jesus was their giant baby.

I also celebrated Hanukkah. We'd light the candles. I'd get the eight gifts. I went to Jewish preschool and learned all the prayers. I spun the dreidels and tore open the gelt and ate my latkes with sour cream and applesauce.

And I'm a damn lucky kid for being able to experience both. Damn lucky. I always felt that way. Imagine, an only child with eight days of Hanukkah followed by Christmas at like 5 different houses? I'd make out like a bandit.

Hanukkah was fun, but Christmas was an event. An early morning wake up for presents at our place. Then we'd speed over to Carlos's house with *café con leche* and *pastelitos* and open presents there. Next stop, my best friend LeeAnn's house. My mom would chat with hers while she and I compared all our gifts. I got a Tamagotchi, she got a GigaPet. How many Beanie Babies did Santa bring you? From there, it was off to lunch at Mimi and Papa's. More *café con leche*, more *pastelitos*. *Croquetas*. Little blue tins of cookies spread around the house. Materva and Jupiña, flowing like wine. Then we'd head to Alina's house. She was my mom's best friend from Cuba. I grew up with her kids; her son might as well have been my brother. We'd run around the house with all our new toys, hyped up on inordinate amounts of sugar and eventually crash. My dad would carry me to the car, we'd drive home and wake up on December 26. Back to life. Back to reality.

You see, because my husband is Israeli and Jewish, my kids are already getting that part of my story. They're going to the same Jewish preschool I went to. They sing the same prayers over the candles on the menorah. They, too, run feverishly around their uncle's house looking for a piece of matzos while their older cousins text their friends about what cool after-party to go to. I'm not missing out on sharing that part of my story, because it's so similar to my husband's. But I want to share my whole story with them. The part my husband was never a part of, doesn't understand, and never experienced in his own life. We owe it to our kids to give them the full story of where they come from.

//

That part of my story, the loud Cuban parties and Christmastime extravaganza, seemed to come to an end at some point in my early twenties.

Carlos, my mom's business partner, died in 2011. My mom's mom, Mimi, died the following year. For some reason, she lost touch with her friend Alina. And LeeAnn and her family moved to Orlando. Our giant, happy Christmas spectacle was no more.

To top it off, my mom finally took down the tree after about 15 years. She says it's because Jonah, my younger stepson, was asking her about it. She knew how my husband felt about Christmas, and she didn't want it to be a problem. So she took it down. I told her no one asked her to do that. But she did it. I guess it was time, though. It was the last bit we were hanging onto. The last bit of a time that we couldn't get back.

//

It's like being homesick for a time, more than a place. It's feeling like a thread in the fabric of your identity is being tugged and unraveling, and you're desperately trying to stop it. It's a fear of losing yourself.

As I write this, I think about my husband. And that little elf toy. And what he must be clinging to. Some part of his story that maybe

I don't fully know, a time he might have forgotten or doesn't realize he misses. A time before he rejected Judaism. Before he declared himself an atheist. Before he fought with his dad about Zionism. Before he told his mom he'd rather not join her at synagogue. Before he'd scoff at observant Jews for being brainwashed.

Before he felt this way about being Jewish, there was a time that being Jewish was everything he was. And maybe that time meant more to him than he's remembering. And maybe that's why he's holding on to this elf argument as strongly as I am.

Maybe.

Maybe we're all secretly clinging to something. Maybe that something is our truest self. That little kid, looking up at the big world, saying yes with a big smile. Maybe that's why we'll always feel homesick for a time that's already past, because we miss being that little kid. We forget that they're still there inside of us. We forget that they're the spark of light, guiding us where we need to go. We just need to get in touch with them.

My Papa Hector used to always say I had a star guiding me. That I'd always get what I wanted in life, I'd always be protected, because of my star. When I got pregnant, I truly believed that the baby growing in my belly was that star. That she'd been up there my whole life guiding me and now she was coming down to join me.

Today, I look in my daughter's eyes and see the entire universe swirling around those deep, bright blue marbles. And I know it's her. I'm convinced she's my sister, one of the miscarriages my mother had before me. My star sister. And just like she's been guiding me all this time, she's continuing to guide me now. Subtly reminding me how to tap back into my truest self and how to take care of myself when I lose touch with my little voice. She triggers all of the memories from my past I've forgotten are essential pieces of patch-work connecting the fabric that is my whole self. The closer I get to putting those pieces together, the closer I get to finding that elusive mental peace. The mental peace of a carefree child experiencing the world without filters. The big sigh followed by the bigger grin. The lightness. The peace. It's still there, inside all of us. Time hasn't stolen it. Mark Zuckerberg hasn't stolen it. The lizard kings haven't stolen it. It's just become harder to access because our minds are so crowded with the noise of modern life.

Mental peace is available to all of us. We just need to learn how to... Marie Kondo our inner worlds, if you will.

Chapter 4: Startled

I have been numbing myself to run away from my anxiety and other uncomfortable emotions for most of my life. When I was younger, I would *literally* numb myself by submerging my head in a large kitchen pot of ice water, holding my breath for as long as I could, because it seemed like the only relief from the massive migraine swelling my brain against my skull.

The numbing manifested in lots of ways. The ice water, of course, is the most literal example. But I would also lash out. I had a terrible temper. I'd scream at my friends, at my parents. Looking back, those outbursts were my way of throwing whatever uncomfortable emotion I didn't want to feel out at them. I didn't want to and, more importantly, didn't know how to sit with them. Process them. Cope.

Each numbing tactic was a different form of self-soothing. I've collected a few strategies in my fucked-up tool kit of unhealthy coping mechanisms over the years. I would drink to numb. I would have sex to numb. I would purge. I would cut.

The first time I got drunk comes to my mind with the rosy filter of innocence and nostalgia. It was sweet and fun and youthful. I was fourteen, maybe fifteen. A couple of my girlfriends met up with a couple of my guy friends. The guys brought some beers. We met at a park behind an elementary school in the middle of the night. Each mid-pubescent boy lumbered toward us carrying a forty-ounce bottle of Olde English wrapped in a brown paper bag. We each took turns holding our noses and taking a big swig before passing the giant glass bottle off to the next person. We laughed and played games and got silly. It was fun. And after that, I maybe drank another handful of times. A friend's folks would go out of town and they'd have people over. I'd find the sweetest sugary beverage to drink—my calling card was cotton candy vodka with Dr. Pepper.

I liked how it felt, being drunk. It felt like an escape. Like the constant noise inside my head got shushed. My intrusive thoughts would go quiet and I could just be.

I didn't start binge drinking with the intent of blacking out until my second year of college. Before that, I was still dating my high school boyfriend. I used to think he didn't like it when I'd go out and party with my friends. He was insecure. Jealous, even. But, looking back and recalling that memory as I write this, maybe that wasn't super accurate. Maybe I was insecure. I didn't trust myself. I was afraid of having too much fun. I was afraid of getting into trouble. I was afraid of wrecking things. Either way, I spent most of freshman year locked away in my dorm room studying, which wasn't the worst thing because I got straight A's that year and was able to enter into my major a year early to get started on the classes I was most interested in.

//

Back in high school, I had a huge crush on my best guy friend, Alex. I always used to lie to him and say I needed a ride home from school. I didn't. I just wanted more time with him. Even while I was dating my high school boyfriend, who eventually dumped me after freshman year of college, I had a crush on Alex.

One time, in high school, Alex and I went to our friend's house for a small party. We all got drunk off Kahlúa. It was disgusting. A few people got sick. We were in the guest house of her grandparents' place, and they caught us and kicked us out. I didn't want to go home because I told my parents I was sleeping over her house. I probably could've just gone home. He could've, too. But we didn't.

Instead, Alex and I drove to a nearby lake and parked the car. Turned the windows down. Played some music. And just sat together. We always enjoyed being close, just being together. Always finding ways to be together.

We stayed there until the sun came up. We spent the entire night together, just sitting side by side, feeling the warm air sweep through the open windows of his navy blue Volkswagen Golf. Hearing the sound of it moving through the trees, with the radio turned down low so the music sounded muffled. The beautiful sound of silence between two people enjoying each other's company.

It'll always be one of my fondest memories from that time. I don't even remember what we talked about. If we even talked. I just remember being with him, and how good I felt. And that "How's It Going to Be" by Third Eye Blind was playing. And when I recall the memory now, and understand what that song is about, and I think about how it all ended up, it makes sense. Everything always makes sense later, right?

How's it going to be. When you don't know me anymore. How's it going to be.

After that night, we just kept on doing our thing, being close friends. Whenever one was single, the other wasn't. It went on like that throughout high school and into the first year of college. Until we both came home from freshman year, and we were both newly single—we finally had the chance to be more than friends. And we let it happen.

It was everything I hoped it would be. I was dating my best friend: I was in love with my best friend. And he was in love with me. All those years and we finally got the thing we both wanted. It was like the final scene from that episode of The Office when Jim doesn't take the job in New York and instead comes back and asks Pam on a date. The excitement on Pam's face after Jim says, "It's a date". **That** feeling. That feeling is what blanketed that entire first bit of time with Alex. Excited love.

But excitement, like most things, is fleeting. Adrenaline doesn't last. Butterflies fly away. And summers end.

We spent the next two and half years dating long distance. He was in school in northern Florida and I was in school in central Florida. We visited each other as often as we could and spent lots of time on the phone. Eventually, we started settling into our own individual lives. Our own friends. Our own schedules. Our own parties. Our own Facebook photo albums. And the distance started getting louder. Like someone turned the volume up on it and I could feel it rattling through my body, shaking my bones.

That feeling triggered me. We can't control distance. We can't control that people grow apart. We can't control much. And that lack of control triggered my anxiety. I only understand this now, though. In the moment, I had no idea why I felt the way I felt. I convinced myself something had to be wrong with me. He never felt that way. He wouldn't stay up all night crying because he missed me or couldn't reach me. He wouldn't become frozen with fear, thinking I was hanging out with my ex. He wouldn't obsess over photos I was tagged in. He wouldn't cry. He wouldn't spiral. So obviously, I was the problem. Something was wrong with me. I always thought everyone lived in constant dread, debilitated by intrusive thoughts and worry, just like I did. It wasn't until I spent this chunk of my life with someone who didn't experience any of these things that I started to connect the dots. I kept making appointments for therapy and cancelling them, talking myself out of the idea that maybe I needed help. Until, of course, I finally had no choice.

//

When I was getting ready to graduate college, I had no idea where I was going to end up. I knew where I wanted to end up, where I was *supposed to* end up, where society had taught me I should want to end up, but I couldn't imagine how I was going to get there. I couldn't see it or feel it. It was intangible. And that scared me. It made me anxious and I started to freak out. That initial freak out was the catalyst that thrust me into the twisting and turning journey that I've since learned is called my twenties.

I always wanted to move back to Miami, live in my grandparents' beach condo, and work at the ad agency I had interned for. That was **the plan**.

But I couldn't see how to accomplish it. The opportunities hadn't presented themselves yet, so I couldn't see how I would be able to make that happen. I always want to know what's going to happen next, to control it. And since I couldn't put my hands on that goal and control it and make it happen, I did what I could with what I had to ease my anxiety. I consumed myself with someone else's goals—my boyfriends goals.

Alex's goals were different from mine. And at the time, they seemed more attainable, more tangible. I became obsessed with controlling his next step, pretending like I could decide for him. He wanted to graduate and move to Arizona and study to become a national park ranger. This option didn't fit **the plan**. He also suggested he might move to Miami with me, live in my grandparents' condo, and wait on tables while I pursued my career in advertising. Looking back, he only offered up that second option to placate me. To shut me up and ease my anxiety. He was never going to move back to Miami. He never wanted to follow me back here and watch me pursue my dream while completely throwing his out the window. And that I thought he would just showed how naive and blind I was. Whether it was by love or by anxiety or by fear, I was blind. Blind to reality.

Well, soon enough reality began to rip away that blindfold and present itself.

//

I was home alone, the entire day free of any sort of responsibility. No class. No work. No worries. I woke up and took my friend's dog Knox for a walk. I was puppy-sitting him for her while she was at class. I walked him up and down the back lot of my college apartment complex. The weather was perfect. As I walked the dirt path, the air was electric, the bushes buzzing from the breeze rustling through their leaves. The trees were noisy with little families of chatty birds and skittish squirrels.

Knox pulled at my arm, rushing me. But I felt so still. I could hear every bird chirp and every squirrel claw at the bark. Surrendering to the moment, I tilted my head back, closed my eyes and let the sun warm my face. I saw orange and felt a warm wind cradle my shoulders. Knox kept yanking at his leash as he tried hurrying forward, not knowing where he was going or what was in front of him. And I remember thinking, *I want to be more like Knox. I want to be so eager and fearless that I rush forward, tugging at the leash that is the present and race into the future with a vigor and force.* And then I stopped, realizing I was idolizing and admiring a dog and quickly laughed myself back into the moment.

I went back upstairs to my apartment, unhooked Knox from his leash and followed him into my bedroom. I had left my phone upstairs that whole time. I had a missed call, from my boyfriend Alex. He rarely called. I immediately felt the rush of excitement as I tapped his name to call him back. I was eager to tell him all about my morning, about walking Knox and the weather and the birds. Tell him how happy and peaceful I felt. He probably wouldn't care all that much, but for some reason that never stopped me. He had become distant, but I still shared all my thoughts with him. Maybe because somewhere deep inside I hoped that eventually he'd start caring again, like he had at the beginning. But alas, our boat had developed its very own slow leak.

He answered. His tone was flat. Was he happy, upset, annoyed? I couldn't get a read on him. Three years of dating and I just couldn't get a read on him.

The conversation is kind of a blur. I remember bits and pieces. "You know how I've been feeling kind of down lately?" "I can't figure out what I want to do with my life and you already know exactly what you want to do." "I need to be on my own." "Without." "You."

I felt my heart just dry up. I felt like my blood stopped pumping. And I was soaking wet. I just remember being soaking wet. I broke out in a cold sweat, instantly. It was as if every pore all over my skin opened up and started crying. And my eyes did the same. My entire body was crying. Sobbing. Heaving. Trying to make sense of what was happening. It was all so unexpected. Like someone just walked up to me, smiled and swung a gigantic slab of wood at my face. It stung.

I remember telling him I was sorry. I remember denying him at first. Justifying why we should remain together. Desperately piecing together rationalizations of how we could make it work, clinging to the fantasy. I told him I didn't want to stop talking to him. That I couldn't because I loved him so much. I couldn't imagine my life without him. My brain couldn't process it. I was so drained, like someone had sucked my soul out of my belly button with a vacuum cleaner. I was just shriveled up on the bed, wet with grief, my mouth somehow making words that landed into the receiver and onto his ears. I remember saying goodbye. He said, "This isn't goodbye. We're still going to talk. You can always talk to me."

And I know what I said. I know I told him that I wasn't going to be able to do that. I wouldn't be able to talk to him because it would hurt too much. Leaving the wound open would deny the healing process. I knew that and I'm glad I was able to say that to him and explain myself. Because as soon as that phone call ended, we ended. It was over. I shut and locked the door to the six years before. The six years of meeting him, getting to know him, falling in love with him, hating him, wanting him, loving him, desperately loving him, falling deeper and deeper in love with him until I was completely consumed. It swallowed me whole. I didn't know anything but loving him. I would've done anything for him, anything he asked. And with a phone call, he became my past.

//

Hanging up that phone was impossible. I couldn't bear to accept that it was over, that he was gone and out of my life. The door to my room was closed and as my lungs struggled for breath, I imagined the four walls inching closer to me. The grief was suffocating. But, as the dust and rubble of the demolition of my reality began to settle, my vision suddenly became overwhelmingly clear. For a split second I was able to see through the moment, witness the flicker of insight I was meant to gather from it. It disappeared as instantly as it came, but although I couldn't articulate what it was just then, it led me to take a very specific inspired action. I went to go see a therapist. Right then, just a few hours after hanging up with him.

I remained in therapy for the last few months of college, and I've been seeing therapists semi-regularly since then. To be honest, I only spent one session sifting through my emotions surrounding the breakup. I came to terms with it rather quickly and embraced my new reality. The bulk of my therapy dealt with everything besides my relationship. I explored my past, my family, my blocks, my insecurities. Things I would have never given myself the time to reflect on. This was also the first time I had ever been given a word to catch all the mental baggage I had been dragging around with me for the past two decades. The word was anxiety. It was as if my therapist handed me a pair of glasses with the right prescription and I could finally see the world around me clearly for the first time.

Through this messy unpacking process, I was able to come out the other side with a stronger understanding of myself. I see now that it was an integral part of my story, a necessary step that carried me into the following chapter of my life.

//

I had been flirting with the idea of going to therapy during those last few trying months of our relationship. I denied, desperately, that anything could be wrong with us, convincing myself that I must be the problem. *He is a great boyfriend, he loves me, supports me, inspires me. How could I possibly be unhappy? Something must be wrong with me.* I always found a reason not to go. But as I sat on the floor of my college apartment, among the shattered pieces of my old life, I couldn't come up with a good enough reason not to.

My school offered free counseling on campus. I went and sat in a small waiting room lit with fluorescent lighting too bright for my bloodshot eyes. After about forty-five minutes of sitting alone in that room, periodically forcing myself to acknowledge the reality that this did in fact just happen, a young man with rimless glasses and wet hair finally came to escort me into an even smaller room. This room was lit with just a lamp, a love seat nestled against the wall. I sat on it alone, facing him, the cushions hugging me. I curled my legs up and wrapped my arms around them, making myself as small as possible. The only comfort I felt was in the plush embrace of that blue suede sofa.

I had never spoken to a therapist before. I can only describe the experience as ripping off all your skin while simultaneously taking a warm bath. I ripped myself bare, divulging all the intimate, gory details of the last few hours. But as I sat there, exposed and vulnerable, he soothed me with just the right words and questions, leading me to my answers. He did have to ask the mandatory questions. Why was I there, was I going to hurt myself, was I going to hurt someone else. He couldn't believe the break-up had just happened. I don't remember much else of the session besides him continuing to pass me boxes of Kleenex.

Afterward, I had to sit at a computer and fill out my intake form. A slew of questions about my background and health and lifestyle. I think it asked me three different times for my relationship status. Each time I winced from the vicious irony, clicking the little bubble next to the word "single."

One question asked me whether or not I startled easily. I glazed by it, marking no, and moved on to the next string of questions about my family history. A few questions later I nearly fell out of my seat. Someone opened the door next to me to enter the room and I was so startled I jumped, my heart racing in my chest. After taking a few breaths, I huffed a sarcastic laugh to myself and scrolled back up a few questions.

"Do you startle easily?"

Yes.

Chapter 5: A New Mental Illness

"If you are depressed you are living in the past.
If you are anxious you are living in the future.
If you are at peace you are living in the present."
—Lao Tzu

Anxiety is fear of losing control. Your brain tricks you into believing you can control everything outside of yourself. And when that doesn't happen (spoiler alert: it never does), you begin reacting out of fear.

Fear of falling behind (looking back on your life and thinking you should be farther ahead.)Fear of losing control (of the future, and all your grand plans.)Fear of missing out (on everything everyone else is doing, right now.)

I can't help but feel like none of us are really living in the present. We're so busy consuming everyone else's present moment and manufacturing our own in order to keep up, that our truly present moments are just passing us by. It's like a whole new level of mental illness that we don't quite have a name for yet.

//

"So, what brings you in today?"

She's about my age. Blonde hair, blown dry, flowing past her shoulders. Her name is Lauren, too. That's one of the reasons I chose her to be my therapist. Somehow that gave her an extra credential that the other candidates on FindYourTherapist.com didn't have. Her last name was the same as the town I grew up in. Extra points, again.

"Well, I just suffered my first panic attack and I think I have some stuff to work out."

I'm contorted into a pretzel on her office sofa, unconsciously digging my nails into a pillow with some inspirational quote stitched into it.

"Have you been to therapy before?" she asks, routinely.

Not since my college boyfriend ripped my guts out over the phone, sending me to spend my last few months of college visiting the onsite counselor twice a week to dig through the enormous baggage I'd brought with me into my adult life. We barely unzipped that oversized and overstuffed bag before college ended and I had to move back home. I never thought to find another therapist until now. Three years later. On the other side of my first panic attack.

"Yes, I briefly saw a therapist in college," I mumble into my hair.

//

It's 2 a.m. and my body is jolted awake without warning. My heart is banging against my chest faster than I've ever felt it bang before. My breath is sneaking out of my lungs as if it's army crawling under barbed wire. I'm nauseous. Confused. Terrified.

I wait a few minutes to see if I can just breathe myself out of it, but eventually I have to wake my fiancé and ask for help. He has a heart rate monitor on his phone. I press my finger against it and wait. 170 bpm. That's beats per minute. For context, a normal resting heart rate should be around 60–100 bpm.

My thoughts raced.

Okay, so I'm dying. I am having a heart attack and I am dying.

Turns out I may have overreacted, because after a quick trip to the nearest Urgent Care Center and being hooked up to an EKG machine, I was told I had just had a panic attack. Heart palpitations was the clinical term.

Heart palpitations.

I woke up from a sound sleep with…heart palpitations.

Why?

Why, indeed.

I wish I knew. I wish I could put my finger on it and be like, *Yep, that was it. That one thing really threw me for a loop that day and got me so worked up that I woke myself up with a panic attack.*

But, I can't. The day was perfectly uneventful.

In that moment—the one where I was clutching at my chest and gasping for breath in the middle of the night, searching for answers-—I couldn't think of a single thing that could have caused it.

And therein lies the problem. Assuming one single thing caused it.

But, first, let's backtrack. Before the fiancé. Before the panic attack. Before all of that, I was just a regular twenty-three-year-old girl, thinking a few therapy sessions and a bachelor's degree qualified me to be a fully functioning adult.

Being twenty-three is a funny time. You really think you've got it all figured out, don't you? Fresh out of college, the whole world at your fingertips. Until you stop to look around one day and realize... now what?

As long as I can remember, I always had an answer to that question. I had a plan for the next step. I knew where I wanted to end up, or where I was told I should want to end up, and I did what I needed to do to get there. You see, young women get to subscribe to one of two life paths. You can be a mother, or you can have a career. Never both. We can dig into why that is later. But for now, I bring it up to offer context. I chose the career path. I was going to be independent and self-sufficient and successful on my own. I was never going to get married or have kids. People did that for all the wrong reasons and I wasn't going to fall into that trap.

That was a really nice story, until it wasn't. Until I found myself working at a job and having no idea what was next for me. For the first time in my life I didn't have a plan or a goal to work toward. I had spent the last twenty-three years going to school, taking tests, submitting applications, applying to internships, and coveting job titles until finally I landed exactly where I was supposed to. I had gotten all things on my list. I got the degree. I got the job. I even got my beach condo. A perfect dismount, sticking the landing. And after throwing my hands up and looking around at the crowd to bask in my achievement, I finally caught my breath and crumbled under the weight of a crushing realization: *I don't want to be here. I don't want to do this.*

My early twenties were underlined by a distinct fear of always being late for something. Like I was rushing to get to some destination, but not knowing where it was. I didn't even know if I wanted to go there.

We're shown what our life and path is supposed to look like and we expect to get it. To want it. We're made to feel like we should know what we're doing. Like we should have our shit together. And at twenty-three years old, I didn't. Not even a little bit. I roamed around with all these grand ideas racing inside my brain; ideas of how I could be happy, fulfilled, contribute to society. I chased them, trying to see where they might lead; it left me dizzy and confused. It left me not knowing what I wanted, if I was happy, if I should be doing what I was doing, or if I even knew how to do what I was doing.

All of these intangible ideas floated around in my brain, acting like helium that filled my head up like a balloon until I felt like my feet were lifting from the ground.

I was just floating around, trying to get a grip.

And being in your twenties feels exactly like that—like being a balloon. We're full of hot air, floating around in space with no real destination or purpose. Someone pumped us up with these ideas of grandeur—college, career, money, success, stability, family—and then they tied it up with a nice little bow called a diploma and let go. They sent us out into the real world, with no intention or direction, and we're supposed to figure it out. Which is fine, we're a resilient bunch. We can handle it. But I wish someone had prepared us for the feeling of aimlessness that comes with post-grad life. It's like no one wanted to admit how bleak it would be. Graduating into a nearly jobless market, being forced to move back in with our parents, realizing we don't want to spend the rest of our lives doing what we just devoted the past four years of our lives studying—why weren't we prepared?

My millennial generation has been fed a recipe for success, a vision of what life is supposed to look like, based on a dated generalization from generations past. So we graduated and got out into the world with this anxious feeling to pursue "success." We had no idea what success was, and that made us feel like we were doing something wrong.

It's causing an anxiety epidemic. We feel like we're supposed to be doing something, but aren't exactly sure what it is. We're treading water while playing a gigantic game of Marco Polo, desperately trying to chase after success. We are told we are supposed to work hard and make money; but no one ever taught us why. Why should we be working so hard? Just for money? Just to fit into this vague definition of success? We were never once made to sit down and ask ourselves what would make us happy. And isn't that all success really is—being happy with your life?

Finding success may be as easy as opening our eyes and putting our feet down, realizing we've been in the shallow end all along.

Success is intangible, and it is unique to each individual. Success takes time and experimentation and risks. Success requires finding the recipe that tastes the best to you. We know how to solve differential equations and pass standardized tests and write annotated bibliographies, but we don't know what we want! We just know what we are supposed to want. And that mental dissonance is causing us anxiety. Causing us to feel like we're forgetting something, missing something.

For four years I tirelessly prepared for the future. For four years I was trained to want a certain outcome. I picked a major. Worked hard, studied, read, lost sleep, studied some more. I followed the dotted line to success. I was told if I worked hard and graduated I would find a job in this field that I had devoted the past four years to learning. I would "succeed." That was the plan. But from my own experience, and my conversations with my fellow post-grads, I began to see that plan unraveling. The smoke and mirrors faded away and we started seeing that plan for what it really was: a cop out. It was a shoddy instructional manual to happiness passed down from the generation before us. It worked for them, so it should work for us. But no one took the time to craft a new manual for us, one that fits our generation. So now we're left to figure it out ourselves and we're seeing the cracks in the system.

As millennials, we grew up surrounded by innovation. We are a generation that saw the birth of the internet, smart phones, social networking. We've witnessed social norms crashing down around us: gay rights, drug reform, a black president! It is ingrained in our system to try to test limits, push boundaries, and fight the status quo. We are obsessed with change. It has been estimated that we will have fifteen to twenty jobs over the course of our working lives! Why? Not because we are lazy, flighty, or entitled. Because we aren't willing to settle. We want to make a difference and an impact on the world. We are creators, innovators, thinkers, speakers, and believers, and it's time for our balloons to land.

//

Age really is just a number. I learned this to be abundantly true after meeting and getting to know a man named Gani. One would think we wouldn't have much in common. He's thirteen years my senior, divorced with two kids, a mortgage, a business, an understanding of what "taxes" are. When I met him, I was twenty-three-years-old, working at my first post-grad job, living the single life, and frequenting too many happy hours. My responsibilities were scarce, my social life was thriving, and I was utterly unattached. We were two different people. So you'd think, until you heard our stories.

Around the same time that I started dating Alex, Gani had just gotten married. His is not my story to tell, so I'll only say in general terms what my take on it is. I believe as we near the age of thirty, we begin to panic. We see friends and peers hitting all the milestones, getting married and having babies, and begin experiencing that perpetual feeling of being late to something, like we've missed the train and don't know if another is ever coming.

So, what happens? We jump on the next train and hope it's taking us where we need to go.

Sometimes, that train takes us far away from our destination. Sometimes, it takes us exactly where we were hoping to go. And, even still, sometimes we decide on a different destination once we've already gotten aboard.

I believe this is what happened to Gani's marriage. They jumped on the train thinking it was the right one and only realized later that it wasn't taking them where they needed to go. Before either of them could realize or articulate this to each other, they got pregnant. A joyous occasion, of course, but also a surefire way to stay on the wrong train. Adding a baby to the mix only intensifies the speed of the train, reminding its passengers that it has no plans of stopping.

So, rather than get off, they stayed the course. They remained married, had baby number one and followed it up with baby number two to keep him company. Because that's what we do when we can't find the exit. We hunker down where we are and hope for the best. We convince ourselves that we can get used to the circumstances, even if they aren't ideal. And, just like I experienced in my past relationships, we excuse shortcomings in order to force life to fit our plans, in order to convince ourselves that we are on the right train.

I was kindly escorted off of my train with a quick, yet painful breakup. Gani's exit wasn't as easy.

You see, while I was dealing with the aftershock of that fateful phone call, and the therapy sessions that followed, Gani was simultaneously seeing his marriage for what it really was for the first time. He had to remove the blindfold and face reality. He had to do it with his marriage, I had to do it with myself in therapy, we all have to do it because it is part of the human experience. We can't help but get caught up and let our wants and desires get carried away into fantasies that we willingly convince ourselves to be reality. We make plans upon plans with no basis in the present moment, and fool ourselves into thinking they'll matter one, five, ten years down the line.

After his divorce, much like after any loss, Gani did some soul-searching. He took stock in his life, saw it for what it really was, and adjusted accordingly. He took comfort in knowing he'd always have the unconditional love of his two boys. He accepted his future as a single father. He promised himself he would never date. Dating was not going to be a part of his plan.

As they say, "We plan. God laughs."

To be fair, he did stick to his plan to some degree. He didn't date. All the women he had become serious with in his past, including his ex-wife, were relationships that blossomed out of friendships. And after his divorce, he didn't date. Gani's first date with me was the first first date he had ever been on.

Of course, I had done my fair share of dating by then. By the time I had met Gani, I had been single for a few years and dating apps were just becoming popular. Tinder literally turned dating into a sick and twisted virtual slot machine and it totally crippled my generation when it came to building meaningful and lasting relationships. To say I was jaded about entering into a relationship with someone would be an enormous understatement.

Toward the end of 2013, I had sworn off dating altogether. I deleted all of my dating apps, and my social media apps too. A few months after this dramatic purging, a few friends talked me into going to a concert for a band I had never heard of. A cute guy came up to me as I watched from the back of the venue, leaning up against the bar. We hit it off and I gave him my number. The next day, he asked me out.

"I felt like we had a connection," he texted.

I immediately rolled my eyes at that, thinking of all the men before him who had sent me similar sentiments, only to ghost me after getting what they wanted. But, there she was again. That friendly nudge in my belly. That little voice assuring me it was safe.

With some hesitation, I typed back, "Maybe there was a little bit of a connection," and agreed to go on a date.

That first date served as the impetus for the following years of more dates, getting to know each other, and eventually falling in love.

And one insight strikes me most when I reflect on how similar our experiences were before we met, considering how far apart they feel on the timeline of life. That insight is this: The person you are going to end up with is out there becoming the person you are going to end up with.

Maybe we aren't as in control as we think we are. We aren't in control of who we are becoming, we just become it. And look back later and are able to put the pieces together for the map that got us here.

Chapter 6: First Comes Love

H*e kissed me! He kissed me, he kissed me, he kissed me!*
That is what's going through my head as I hop around in the elevator waiting to get off on my floor. That was *the* best first date I've ever been on! And I have been on **a lot** of first dates. Not too many second dates, definitely no thirds. But of the many first dates I've sat through, this one left a serious impression.

The elevator doors open and I scuttle my shaky knees toward my door. I'm literally skipping my way down the hall, my heels clacking around beneath me. I dance my way through the front door, disrobing as I lock it behind me. I'm down to my bra and underwear and I do one final celebratory dance before throwing myself onto my giant king-sized bed in pure joy.

I'm giddy and giggling like a little schoolgirl. I have consciously given myself permission to enjoy this moment. Savor it. Because I know it's fleeting. Every decent first date comes with that high. The buzzy butterflies. The eager anticipation. Will he call? Did he like me? What pattern of china will we choose? I know better than to get my hopes up.

But in the back of my head I understood something. In the pit of my stomach I felt something stir. A spark of connection. A knowing that something bigger was unearthing itself. I didn't know what or how or when. But I know it made me feel happy and nauseous at the same time. So I choked it back with the leftover tofu pad Thai I brought home from our date and washed it down with some stale wine from the previous week.

Don't check your phone, he didn't text, he's still driving, don't check your phone.

I knew this particular sense of disappointment all too well. Years of dating taught me never to expect them to follow up.

Don't check it, don't check it, don't check it.

So I went to bed. I shimmied my way beneath my comforter and yanked the metal chord hanging from the fan to turn out the light. I lay my head on the pillow and closed my eyes.

Maybe he texted you. He probably texted you. You should check. What if he did and you don't answer and he thinks you don't like him.

Dammit!

So I grabbed my phone and swiped it open with a hesitant finger and a defeated cringe closing my eyes.

"Hey Lauren. I had such a great time tonight. I hope we can do it again. You're probably sleeping, but I hope you have sweet dreams. Good night."

Insert blank stare textured with compulsive blinking. Followed by stupid, giant, cheesy smile. Ear to ear and back again.

//

That next Monday morning at work, I was itching to tell someone about my date. I had already spilled my guts to every girlfriend who would listen. Going into every gory detail from what I wore, to the way the light hit his face, to all the reasons why we're probably soul mates. But when I got to work I was dying to keep talking about this epic first date.

After college I landed the exact job I wanted, at a small creative ad agency in Miami that I interned with my freshman year of college. I did everything in my power to make that job happen, and it did.

Now, with that being said, I started that job with little to no experience. I was hired to shadow the existing Account Executive. Come to find out, about a month in, she was moving to LA. Not only was she my mentor, the one I had been learning from day in and day out, but she was also one of the only other women in the company. There was one other and she was the wife of our other, more senior, account executive.

So, to catch up, I started this job as a super green twenty-two-year-old, my mentor left, and I was the youngest person (and only girl) in the company.

I remember very distinctly my boss coming up to me after my mentor announced she was leaving. He sat me down and assured me that he believed in my abilities. He let me know he understood how green I was and he knew I'd have a steep learning curve. He believed I could handle it. But then he said this.

"Lauren, this is a sink or swim moment. We're feeding you to the sharks. You can either let them eat you or learn to swim with them."

That was a pivotal moment for me. Up until that point I was quite literally hiding in the shadow of the woman I had been shadowing. I didn't speak up much, too afraid of saying something stupid in front of all those grown-ass men. I kept scrupulous notes, documenting everything I possibly could. Which clients needed more attention, which art director worked faster, how long lunch took, what was everyone eating. By the time my boss handed me this giant stepping stone in my career, I was ready to leap onto it. I knew what the sharks were and I was ready to meet them head on.

From that day forward I started owning my voice. I trusted myself. I spoke up in creative meetings. I shared ideas. I organized my department. I organized the creative department. I showed up.

I showed up that day and I kept showing up every day after that. And over time I earned the respect of all those men. When I spoke, they cared and they listened. And they heard me. And little by little I became a viable member of that family.

I became particularly close to our two art directors because they were nearest to my age. We began going to lunch together, collecting inside jokes and sharing our list of grievances about the company with each other. They became my best friends at work because we spent so much time together. We got in early, we stayed late. We drank beers on the balcony, we held our heads in our hands while we waited for the boss to approve our presentations the night before a meeting with clients. We were tight. And this meant we knew about what was going on in each other's lives. There's only so much time you can pass by bitching about a shitty printer, after all.

We all had pretty different lives outside of work. Arnaud was the hipster other hipsters looked to know what was cool. He was tall, French, and had a handlebar mustache. He enjoyed getting tattoos, combing his beard and the occasional mosh pit. Eric was a big guy with a bigger mouth. At first, he nestled himself deep beneath my skin and everything he said drove me crazy. Over time, though, I warmed up to him and he became one of my closest friends. I, of course, served as endless entertainment to these two men. I was a young, naive white girl looking for my Jewish prince charming as I scoured through Tinder. That agency became home to me. Those coworkers became my big dysfunctional family. I loved them and I trusted them.

//

So, back to the morning after my epic first date. I had gotten into the habit of carpooling with Eric to work every morning, so by the time we got to the office I had already talked his ear off about my enchanted evening. I remember him being very excited for me about going on a date with a "nice Jewish boy." When Arnaud got to work, Eric and I had a pot of coffee going and were starting up our computers for the day. The three of us were the only ones there for a while, so I made sure to fill Arnaud in as we prepared our morning coffee.

"His name is Gani. He picked me up and had the fanciest car! I've never seen a car so fancy. And we ate Thai food which is my fave. You know that! And we talked so much they literally had to kick us out. We didn't realize we were the only ones there. Isn't that crazy?! And when he dropped me back off, guess what happened!"

I was talking a mile a minute, the Cuban espresso shooting through my veins so fast it might as well have been strapped to my arm with a needle. Arnaud sat across from me, his chin resting in his hand, sleepy eyes smiling back at me. "What happened next?" he humored me.

"He kissssed me," I sang to him, doing a little dance in my chair.

"This one is going to be different," I promised. "I'm not going to internet-stalk him. I won't."

They each rolled their eyes around their heads in unison.

"I swear! I'm so over that. I won't obsess. I'll be totally cool."

Social media has led us to falsely believe we have the right to know everything we want about a person, with little to no context.

We make rash decisions based on a narrow slice of life carefully curated as someone's online profile. Intellectually, I know this is wrong. But, it can be hard to fight the urge.

Two days later, I was deep into a full-fledged investigation into this guy. Internet-stalking is my gift and my curse. I'm *too* good at it. I won't bore you with how I got there, but I found myself scrolling through the blog of a lifestyle photographer who shared a photo shoot he had done with my epic first date, his wife and their two children.

And that, my friends, is the sound of the other shoe dropping. Let that sink in.

Arnaud had his noise canceling headphones cradling his ears. I tapped him on the shoulder and he swung them around his neck and turned to me. My face was a mixture of shame and utter defeat. My bubble was effectively burst and I was completely deflated.

"I did something bad." I confessed to him.

"What?" he smirked at me.

"I found him online."

"And…?"

"And…" I drew in one long breath. "And I found out he is married…was married…I don't know. Oh, and he has two kids. I think."

Eric had his back to us but I knew he was listening. He chimed in without even turning in his chair. "Well what did you expect? He's thirty-something years old. It'd be weirder if he wasn't married before."

I mulled that one over for a while. I'd be lying if I said it had never occurred to me. I mean, on our first date, our age did come up. When I said I was twenty-three, he turned so pale I thought he might actually pass out into his bowl of *tom ka gha*. He took a moment to gather himself and responded with a hesitant, "Okay… um…so I'm thirteen years older than you."

Something you should know about me is that mental math is my weakest quality. The calculator in my brain is perpetually out of batteries. As I stared at him, counting my fingers below the table, he continued. "I'm thirty-six."

I was surprised. He didn't look 36. He looked much younger. That would make him the oldest guy I had ever dated. However, I went on a few dates with a guy a few months before who was only a couple years younger than that, and he had been divorced (technically separated, which I only found out during a Facebook-stalk session.) So I knew that could be an option. But by no means did I assume he *had* to have been married. I mean, my boss was about the same age and was never married. It's not totally bizarre. So my hopeful, naive mind let me believe he was never married, definitely didn't have kids and that our future relationship would go off without a hitch.

Stupid, stupid, stupid.

//

As luck would have it, Valentine's Day fell exactly one week after our first date. We had been talking quite a bit, both of us seemingly interested, but naturally things were still very new, very reserved.

I was at work brainstorming a new campaign with Eric and Arnaud when I received a giant bouquet of flowers at the office. I'd never really received flowers on Valentine's Day. And if I had, it was only after constant pestering and blatant hints on my part. So I wouldn't allow myself to think they could possibly be from Gani. We had only been on ONE date.

The card read, "To the beautiful writer with a beautiful smile. I hope we can stay connected a while."

No name. No signature. I had the tiniest little feeling down in my gut urging me to believe they were from him. But I refused it. I proceeded to call my mom and my best friend to see if they had sent the flowers. They hadn't.

Finally, after calling and failing to reach the busy florist a dozen times to ask who sent me flowers, I sucked it up and asked him.

Not only did he tell me they were from him, but he also went on to apologize. He frantically back-pedaled, going on about knowing we've only been on one date, we're just friends and he just meant he hopes to stay connected in any way, not just romantically, he knows we aren't together, he just thinks I deserve flowers on Valentine's Day, it doesn't matter who they're from. Spewing run-on sentences strung together with nerves, he chaotically tried to cover-up this grand gesture of affection.

It was really sweet. And I felt so relieved, so flattered, and so cared for.

I told him he didn't need to apologize, that I loved the flowers.

"But the florist says you keep calling."

"Yeah, to find out who sent me flowers."

//

I only found out later the stress Gani had put himself through to get me those flowers. He called every florist in town begging them to put an order in for him ... on Valentine's Day. The ones that didn't laugh and hang up on him gave him a very terse "NO!". He finally found the only florist in South Florida that would put one more arrangement together for him and send it over to some girl he barely knew but wanted to stay connected to for a while.

When we finally straightened it all out, Gani and I continued talking via text. Catching each other up on how our weeks had been, planning the date we had scheduled for the next day.

And then I received a very long string of messages that showed up on my phone with a force, as if someone had been carrying a heavy load of bricks in their arms, which finally gave way, dropping the load of bricks at my feet.

It was Gani, shitting bricks.

"I wanted to let you know I just got out of a pretty long relationship…" he sent.

"Okay," I responded, waiting for the rest of the story that I already knew (read: internet-stalking 101.)

"And by relationship, I mean marriage, and by 'got out' I mean divorced."

I didn't tell him I already knew because that would involve me confessing to internet-stalking, which I wasn't ready to do yet.

He then went on to tell me about his kids.

I asked, genuinely not knowing the answer, "So, how many kids do you have?"

"I have six kids," he responded.

My heart sank down to the pits of my stomach, filled up with air and exploded.

"Just kidding, I have two kids."

Ha. Ha. Ha.

"Oh thank god," my fingers responded for me.

I've asked him since if he did that on purpose. To lessen the blow of finding out he had kids. Because when he wrote back saying he only had two kids, I was so relieved. Oh, *just* two. What a relief! When in reality two is still way more than zero.

I definitely came off a lot cooler than if I was learning about all this for the first time. Remember when Phoebe and Joey pretended they didn't know about Rachel being pregnant when Ross told them and they had to fake being shocked? "That is brand new information!" Yeah, it kind of felt like that.

By the time he told me, I had been able to sit with myself and process the possibility of him being divorced with kids. I gave myself the space to really think that through and decide if it felt right and true for me to move forward with a situation like that. Luckily, my voice of intuition tuned out the noise of societal expectation and accepted convention, guiding me toward my decision. A decision I made from a place of truth, not expectation.

Chapter 7: Don't Date and Internet

What ever happened to going steady? People used to date and get to know each other and take the time to discover what they liked about each other. Dating wasn't really like that when I entered the game. Real, meaningful, steady relationships were hard to come by.

After Alex broke up with me, I threw myself into the dating world, at times a bit recklessly. I had never dated before then. I went from my high school boyfriend to dating my high school best friend. I was a total noob.

I experimented with all sorts of ways to meet people: the traditional "meeting a stranger at a bar" to the not-so-traditional "Tindering." But I realized that no matter the avenue, the destination still seemed pretty much the same. Exchange pleasantries, exchange Facebook friend requests, exchange spit, and never hear from each other again.

Why? With things like social media and dating apps, we're simply overstimulated and underwhelmed. There are too many options convoluting our sense of quality and reality. Having too many choices really leaves us with none.

Why have apps like Tinder and Hinge become so popular? Because we have this nearly insatiable need to see what all of our options are and what else is out there. And the apps give us that, pacify that craving just enough. We can flip through a virtual Rolodex of potential candidates, swipe after swipe, until we see something that catches our eye.

On top of that, we crave perfection. We feel entitled to the best there is out there. So when it comes to dating, we often find that reality doesn't match up to our expectations, since we have this irrational expectation of perfection based on false examples of humanity displayed over the internet.

We are constantly bombarded with images of other people's "perfect" lives. Of all the cool things we could be doing with all the cool people we could be friends with. We manufacture this perfectly varnished version of our lives via social media and then feel bad about ourselves when looking in on everyone else's perfectly varnished version of their lives.

It's a vicious cycle and it's causing us to never be satisfied. To always be chasing after something that doesn't exist. How can we be expected to date one person for any length of time when we are constantly craning our necks to look and see who is coming up behind them?

I am a firm proponent of the benefits that social media innovations have given our generation. We are able to share and disseminate information at the click of a button, stay in touch with people from all walks of our lives, network, learn, discuss and explore. It is an amazing tool! But I don't think we have considered the effect it is having on the way we interact with people in real life and the lens we now see life through.

So, when I realized this new guy I was dating was different, I made a promise to myself to date him differently than I had dated others in the past. I decided to step outside the social media bubble and venture into the world of truly getting to know someone. Getting to know him, not his Facebook account. I was on a mission to lift the filters and see how turned on I could really get when I experienced life from the other side of the screen.

//

I didn't become Facebook friends with Gani until four months after we had started dating. In that four months we got to know each other, started a serious relationship, met each other's friends and families, went on trips, fought, made up and took lots of really great pictures. But none of it, not one bit of our relationship, lived online.

This social media abstinence was done intentionally. I entered this relationship knowing I wanted something more serious. And one of the common denominators that I saw affecting my past relationships was the messy layer that social media added to them— the misinformed perception that inherently comes along with judging someone based on the slice of life they choose to share online. It denies partners the intimacy and depth that comes with really getting to know each other. Getting to know all sides of each other's lives, not just the bits and pieces displayed in a news feed.

There are plenty of ways to keep social media from playing third wheel in a relationship, but since most of us aren't ready to go off the grid, here are some ways we can use it to our advantage.

Stalk and Talk

We already know I internet-stalked Gani after our first date. And I discovered all sorts of private information that I didn't need to know yet. It's difficult not to use the technology that's sitting in our hands, and before I knew it, my fingers were traipsing over the keyboard typing his name into the Google search bar. For some reason, we are under the impression that we have the right to know everything about a person immediately. But we forget the consequences of unearthing information that we aren't ready for. It's important to allow a relationship to progress naturally, to trust that our partner will share everything they need to share with us. This way we can keep from jumping to unnecessary conclusions. Let's save that energy and just wait for the bombs to drop, because they usually aren't as detrimental as we think they'll be.

However, there's always a chance that we will find out information about our partners from a third party. Be it overhearing a conversation, glancing at a text message or, as hard as we try to avoid it, stalking their Facebook page. But it doesn't have to lead to distrust. In fact, it can offer a way to start the relationship on a solid foundation of open communication and honesty. For example, I learned Gani may have been divorced with children after our first date. Instead of making a rash decision based on that knowledge, I waited and trusted he would share that information with me when he was ready. And when he did, I was ready to have an honest and compassionate conversation about it.

If we find out something about our partner that we don't like or understand, we should ask them about it. Talk to them. It may be uncomfortable admitting to snooping, even if it was unintentional. But it's more uncomfortable and far more detrimental to any relationship to overanalyze something to the point where the horrible version created in our head stands no chance against the truth.

I'll Show You Mine, If You Show Me Yours

Part of a relationship is sharing where we've come from, who our friends are, and what our lives have been like. One way to do this is by looking back through each other's photo albums. And that's exactly what Gani and I did. Skimming through the events of the past few years, we shared where we'd been, who we were, and why we decided on that particular haircut. Except, rather than a physical photo album, we shared digital photo albums saved forever on our Facebook pages. We showed our Facebooks to each other.

It's undeniable that Facebook is our modern day time capsule. It allows us to document the seemingly best parts of our lives and save them forever, to look back with cringe and nostalgia at all the different times we posed with strangers or wore ill-fitting clothing. But rather than sitting hunched over a laptop scrolling through Facebook pictures blindly taking guesses at who each person is and what their relationship was, why not hear it from the source?

We all have our share of compromising photos we've forgotten about. This gives us a chance to provide context to those photos that may warrant some explanation. Not only will it eliminate the confusion, but it will also serve as an opportunity to become closer and get to know each other better.

Pics or It Didn't Happen

It's hard to fight the urge to post our pictures online because we're being made to believe if we don't post a picture of us enjoying a moment, it never actually existed. We have this compulsive need to share everything we're doing so it's clear what a great time we're all having. And I am not immune to that compulsive need. I wanted to share my relationship because it was new and exciting, and I wanted to make sure I wasn't making it all up! But I knew I wanted to keep it off the internet. So instead, I would text pictures to my few close friends, the ones who would actually care about my happy boyfriend selfies and vacation pictures, and chose to share my relationship with them that way.

You see, sharing is important. Especially when we all live so far away from each other. Eventually friends move across the country, sometimes across the world, and we've become accustomed to using social media to keep in touch. Which is perfectly fine. But there is an alternative to sharing those special and intimate moments with our close friends that doesn't involve posting on a social media site. Starting a group text with close friends is a great way to stay in touch and update each other about what's going on.

Relationships don't work by magic, they take effort. Healthy relationships must start with a strong foundation, one of open communication, understanding, and lots of love. In my experience, eliminating social media from that equation definitely plays a part in keeping that foundation solid. We don't need to post a filtered picture and get likes on Instagram to make a moment real. We don't need to impulsively adjust our Facebook statuses to feel like our relationships are "official." It's been made abundantly clear that social media has changed up the dating game. It's about time we make our own rules for how we play it.

//

Shacking up, playing house, moving in together. It's a topic that seems to have a very specific calculation as to when the timing is right. Like an old family recipe that has to be baked at the exact right temperature for not a second longer than the recipe calls for, or it will burn and ruin Thanksgiving dinner. But our choices are our own and don't fit under one specific recipe. So, how do we know when to start the timer?

I quickly found myself accidentally living at Gani's house. It was closer to my job, his fridge always had food in it, and I happened to have fallen in love with his cat. But mostly, it was because he was there. I hadn't yet committed a toothbrush to his house and my clothes still came back and forth with me in an overnight bag, but yeah, I kind of lived there.

It's something I never gave much thought to when entering into a serious relationship, but it's an inevitable part of the process. It began dawning on me that we were starting to build a life together, but we didn't actually live together. And it was getting a bit tiresome living between two houses. We each had scraps of personal belongings left at each other's places, but we didn't have one place to keep everything. Either he'd forget to pack underwear or I'd forget my make-up bag. But we pressed on.

This all seems like pretty typical relationship behavior. But, as I've learned, there's no such thing as typical. You see, he was currently in the process of buying a new house. And as he was looking for this new house, he couldn't help but include me in the process. We both had every intention of continuing our lives together, so he wanted to know that he was choosing a house that I could also see myself living in. And I felt confident promising that. The thing was, I knew it was what I wanted, but I hadn't considered that I might be presented with this life decision so quickly. I had unknowingly bought into a predetermined time frame; one absent of exceptions or adjustments.

So, I found myself in a situation I would have never thought to prepare myself for. And, since the topic came up, it had me wondering: If I was basically living with him already, why not go all in? I started to realize that my opinions about this had been based solely on accepted convention. There are specific guidelines laid out that we all subconsciously abide by. We're told it's too soon to move in or too late to have kids. We're asked why we are still single or how an engagement can be so long. And we see these conventions perpetuated in our News Feeds all day, every day. But there isn't one universal standard to hold all of our experiences to. Each one is different, with its own unique circumstances. We need to make our decisions based on what's right for us, not what's right for everyone else.

With this in mind, I decided to make my own rules for how I was to go about this transition. More importantly, I reminded myself that I can make my own rules for how I go about most things in life. Just like that little girl in second grade who strung her bangs with beads and had a borderline psychotic collection of Beanie Babies, I didn't give a fuck what was accepted by others. I did what felt good and right for me.

It's important to listen to others who have been there and consider their advice. It's worth trusting those who have our best interests in mind. But the only way to truly know what's right for us is to find out for ourselves. We can't be afraid of making mistakes or falling when we take that leap of faith. We're more resilient than we give ourselves credit for, and from the little I've witnessed in my life, it seems to be worth the fall.

As I closed the door one last time to my tiny one-bedroom beach condo, a space I built for myself alone, I felt overwhelmed with gratitude for all my blessings. Over those few years alone in that apartment I had created a beautiful life for myself and learned from my many mistakes along the way. And suddenly, I had a partner offering to add to that life and make it even bigger and better. It may not be the way I had been told it would happen, it may not be the way it happened for someone else, but I knew it was the right move for me.

Chapter 8: On Purpose

decided I liked this guy enough to give this a try. I didn't know what the future would look like. I couldn't control the outcome. But for the first time, I accepted those universal truths rather than stubbornly deny them. Even more, I embraced them. I was very honest with Gani from the beginning. I let him know that I was serious about him and that I thought we could make it work, and if that ever changed I would make sure to tell him. And so, we embarked on the most profound chapter of either of our lives.

Over the course of six months, I quit my job at the ad agency, I moved in with him and his two sons, we bought a house together, and I became a stepmother. With what seemed like the snap of my fingers, I was suddenly a stay-at-home soccer mom, real housewife of suburbia. I was suddenly domesticated: cooking dinners, shuttling kids to soccer practice, scheduling playdates, cleaning the house, and crafting school projects.

My first internal reaction was to resent all of this. This is not the life I had planned on having. Gani started to ask to take over my bills, reminding me that he ran a successful business and that he could afford to support me.

Support me?! I don't need a man to support me.

I would fight him tooth and nail over every bill he tried to take from me. **Take.** As if he were someone stealing something from me. My independence? My freedom? Maybe. And I wouldn't allow it.

Little by little, I started letting him take over my bills. I found myself for the first time as an adult in a position where I didn't need to work to support myself. It was jarring— I never considered this as an option. And yet, here I was. Financially supported, yet not working for a paycheck.

Of course, I was working. I was working my little butt off trying to prove that I deserved the support he was giving me. Trying to reciprocate it by raising his kids, keeping a clean home, making his life easier any way I could.

All while ignoring that voice screaming up at me from the depths of my being to slow down. To enjoy it. Assuring me I had nothing to prove and reminding me that there was no pressure to be perfect. I could lean into this new life happily and unencumbered by my past hang-ups about what adult life was *supposed* to look like.

Instead, I brushed that voice off with the flick of my broom and kept rage-cleaning the house until it was spotless.

//

First comes love (check), then comes marriage (check), then comes... well you get the picture. Shortly after moving in together, Gani and I made it official and got married. And then shortly after our wedding, we made it super official and got pregnant. As soon as I saw that confirmation on a stick of plastic, dripping with my own urine, everything changed.

That's around the time I started realizing that the work I was doing felt meaningless. After quitting my job at the ad agency and beginning my career as a stay-at-home mom, I had created an online business as a branding coach. I taught my clients (other bloggers and entrepreneurs) how to show up online and brand their own online businesses. In turn, I had to lead by example and do *a lot* of "showing up" online.

But suddenly, I felt that same voice yelling in my ear, telling me to stop. She'd been calmly trying to get my attention for a while, but once I became pregnant, she gave up playing nice and went right to her angry voice. When it came to being online, I felt a resounding *NO*. The pictures of my coffee and the filtering and the hashtagging and the scrolling...it was all bullshit. I suddenly felt a much more meaningful job placed in my hands, and I needed the space to rise to the occasion.

The big realization came to me in one of my weekly therapy appointments. This is the fifth therapist I've seen in my life, including a couple's therapist Gani and I saw together.

I was talking to my therapist about how I'd started losing interest in my work. And I didn't know how to feel about that. I had spent so much time building it and working for it and all I wanted to do was let it go. And then I said it. The one sentence I would have never imagined I would ever say: "I just want to be a mom."

Wait, what?

It seems like over the past few years, I stumbled into my life's purpose without any effort of my own. I became the person I was supposed to be without even trying. I spent so much time in college and in my early twenties reeling about *what I was supposed to be doing with my life*. And all the while, with all that resistance, life figured out how to get me where I was going.

I am meant to be a mom. And a homemaker. And a wife. These are things I would have never imagined in a million years I would be saying. I used to say marriage was an outdated institution that society pressures us into. I used to cringe at the sound of crying babies. I used to pity young mothers who had to give up their careers to stay home and care for their children. I would roll my eyes at the rising divorce rate, as if to say "duh."

But you know what makes me feel like my best self? You know what fills me with purpose? Drives me to be a better person? Lights a fire under my butt? Being a wife and mom.

And it wasn't until I became pregnant with my own child that I was able to admit this. Because up until then, I was "only" a step-mom. And up until then, I felt a void. Because as much as I am a mother to my two boys, as much as I work and sacrifice and teach and nurture them and give everything I have and love them like they're my own...they still have their real mom. They'll always have her. And I'll always be the stepmom. They'll never be able to give me all of their love, not like they give their parents.

They love me, but it's different. And I love them, but it's different. Because it has to be. Because if I gave them my whole heart, I would end up hurt and broken every week they go back to her. Every time they call her mom and me Lauren.

I won't get into the trials and tribulations of stepmotherhood right now, that's another book in itself. But in short, it's all the work of being a mom with half of the satisfaction. I can never give myself over fully to the boys. I can never rip myself open and love them without limits, because I will only end up hurt because they can never do that in return. They have a biological mom who they will always feel that way toward. It'll just always be different. We definitely love each other in a profound and extraordinary way, but we'll always be holding a little something back, because that's just the nature of our situation.

I've never really been able to wear that "mom badge" with pride. Wrap myself in it and make it my identity, even though that's exactly who I've been ever since I stepped into their lives at the ripe age of twenty-three.

As soon as I saw the word "pregnant" pop up on that stick, I felt a shift. All of those years of being a mom but never being able to embrace the role fully. All of those years of sacrificing for the boys and giving to them and loving them. All of those years of being a closeted stay-at-home mom. I could finally come out! I AM A MOM. I'm a really good mom and it is the best job in the world. It is also the most difficult job in the world and soul-crushing at times. But the good outweighs the bad, always.

Chapter 9: Mom Guilt

L ike most moms, I try very hard to be everything for everyone. I never want to disappoint. Especially the kids. It breaks my heart if I ever fall short for them, so I spend a lot of time going above and beyond to proactively compensate.

The same goes for my husband. I never want him to catch me letting anything fall through the cracks. He's accomplished so much with his business, and spends his entire day doing the impossible. So I want him to come home and think I'm doing the same.

I want it to seem like I have it all together, all the time.

The truth is, I'm a fucking mess. He of all people would know that. But I guess I'm still able to fool him. The truth is, I spend a lot of time sobbing into my hands or screaming into my pillow or gritting my teeth so hard I've had to acquire a mouth guard.

It's not easy, man. And no one ever said it would be. But I feel like we're not allowed to admit it—not just to other people, but to ourselves.

Being a parent is really demanding. Making sure they eat. Making sure their food doesn't have bad ingredients in it. Making sure they're making friends, doing homework, passing tests, going to the dentist, developing on schedule, meeting project deadlines, wearing pants.

It's so much. And it never stops. There is no clocking out at the end of the day. I'm always thinking about what everyone else needs, mentally cataloging all of their appointments, meetings, due dates, lessons, parties and whatever else.

Today, we are also encouraged to buy into a cult of perfection-ism that's paraded in front of us online in filtered photos and false narratives about motherhood. It's about time we unsubscribe. Stop watching everyone else be the most perfect mom on Facebook, witnessing women shame each other for how they're raising their children, and reading one article that tells you *this* is the way only to read another to tell you *that* is the way. It's enough to drive anyone insane.

Most days, my needs don't even make it onto the list. And when they do…this happens.

I had been meaning to sign up for this birthing class for a while. But it was on Tuesday nights, which is when the boys have their music lessons. So I had to figure out a sitter. And confirm that my husband could make it home in time Tuesday nights from work.

After watching the task sit on my to-do list week after week, while everyone else's tasks were being crossed off around it, I finally just signed up. I spoke to the teacher on the phone. I put it on my calendar. On the family calendar. Confirmed with the sitter. Set an alarm on my phone.

And then, whoops! The week before, our sitter had a conflict. So I had to bring in reinforcements. I secured my sister-in-law, rescheduled music lessons, made sure my husband would be home on time.

That night, things were going pretty smoothly. We all had dinner together, the boys were having fun with their aunt, things were moving along.

As we were on our way out, it started pouring. Like, *Is there a hurricane we don't know about-* kind of pouring. So we waited a bit, but ended up driving through some pretty bad rain to try and make it to the class on time. Once we're there, we get lost finding the room. A kind janitor finally guided us in the right direction. We walked in ten minutes late. Wet, cold, harried. Everyone goes silent and gives us a confused look.

Turns out our class started the following week. We were in the wrong class, on the wrong day, and I have never been more embarrassed. My husband took it like a champ, laughed it off and we went on our way. I, however, became inconsolable.

This does not happen. I don't mess this stuff up. I am hyper-organized with all of our schedules. I have everyone's appointments and meetings and lessons all logged in chronological order in my brain at all times. I have multiple color-coded calendars filled out at once. This does not happen.

I was so embarrassed. And angry at myself. I couldn't just laugh it off. I had wasted so much time finding a back-up sitter and rescheduling music lessons and rushing my husband home from work. All for nothing.

But my husband, the saint that he is, tried to give me some perspective. He said all the right things that I was not saying to myself. He reminded me that these things happen, we make mistakes and laugh them off and move on. He told me stories of other people who had fucked-up way worse. He hugged me and kissed me and made the best of the situation.

And then, on the drive home, as I continued to cry to myself in the passenger seat, he held my hand and said, "Baby, you're not perfect."

My first reaction was rage. I didn't have time to express it, though, because he immediately followed that statement with: "I wouldn't be with you if you were."

And obviously that made me cry more. Because I put so much pressure on myself to be perfect. For the boys, for my husband, for everyone who needs me. But none of them are asking that of me. No one puts that expectation or pressure on me. I put it on myself.

So the lesson here is, fuck being perfect. It doesn't exist. It's an ideal. I think it's okay to strive for it, and work toward it. Do your best to be your best. But cut yourself some slack every now and then. You'll never *arrive* at perfection. It's not something to achieve. And remember, it's a standard you're holding yourself to, not what anyone else is putting on you.

I'm not going to stop color-coding our calendars and to-do lists. I won't ever like it when the dirty dishes sit in the sink. I'll continue to tout my DYMO label maker around like a concealed weapon. But I'm trying to have a bit more of a sense of humor about it all.

//

Stay-at-home mom. Stay-at-home?! You're so lucky. You get to hang around the house all day in pajamas. You can watch TV and eat snacks and do whatever you want. Nap when the baby naps. Prepare fresh meals. Keep the house clean. Find time for your own hobbies and self-care. Shower. Read. What a dream!

Ha! First I'll say, yes, I am so lucky that I get to stay home. I feel grateful every day, because it's something I *want* to do and I *get* to do it. There are lots of stay-at-home parents who don't have the choice. And lots of other parents who wish they had the choice. And more still who have the choice but would much rather go to work. There is no one right way to do this thing.

Now, that being said, that is NOT how the day of a stay-at-home parent goes down. Like, not at all. I mean the pajamas part is pretty accurate, but that gets old quick. And if you count snacking on leftover applesauce and goldfish crackers a win, then I'm the champ. But most days you just feel like a dog chasing its tail, using up lots of energy to get nowhere. Well, what feels like nowhere. It's easy sometimes to forget that you're raising a little person, who needs you to learn how to function. It can seem like nothing, but it's really everything.

Whether you stay at home or go to work, chances are you put your head down at the end of the night and your brain starts listing off everything you didn't do. I know mine does. I can feel so exhausted and so unproductive all at once. How am I so tired if I didn't do anything all day?

But here's the thing. We DO do things. All day. In those little micro-pockets of time, we somehow get shit done. I don't know how. But we do. We work and we love and we plan and we nurse and we soothe and we teach and we shop and we organize and we clean and we play.

And yet we still feel like we've accomplished nothing. It makes sense when we see everyone online doing every possible thing all at once, forgetting that's a false and filtered fairytale.

I've come to accept that there will always be something on my to-do list that I won't get to. I'll forget to do it. I'll push it off. I'll miss the deadline. I'll need to be reminded more than once. I'll write it down in five different places and still forget. That's just how it's going to be right now.

I'm used to getting things done and being in control and being super dependable and punctual and "perfect." These are things I've wrapped my identity around. And since having kids I am none of those things. BUT I'm a whole slew of other way better, more important things. And that's what matters.

I beat myself up every night that I didn't do enough with my day. But I know that's just not true. I've managed an entire home remodel, a move, family trips, school events, tantrums and attitudes, growth spurts and teething. I've been with the baby, nursing her and teaching her and loving her. I've managed to write an entire book somehow. I have no idea how or when that happened. But somewhere in between all the nothing I was doing, I wrote an entire book. That's gotta count for something, right?

What I'm trying to say is, don't forget those little moments throughout the day where you figure out how to get the things done. Maybe not all the things. But things, nonetheless. And they matter. And you matter. And you wrote a whole book with a baby attached to you and that's a feat in and of itself. Even if no one reads the damn thing. That's something to be proud of. (Maybe that last part was directed just at me.)

Let's stop being so dang hard on ourselves. Drop the guilt. Drop the pressure. And just enjoy these little magical micro-moments. Live in them. Breathe them in. Soak them up. Even when they feel super challenging.

Try to keep that perspective in your back pocket to call upon when you need it. These moments are very temporary and we're going to miss them. The moments where the baby wakes up early from her nap and you didn't get to finish that post and you rock her on your shoulder as you finish it up and send it out. You'll forget about that moment. You'll put your head down at the end of the day and you won't think of it. You'll only think of everything you missed. All the things you did wrong. The moment you lost your temper or the deadline you forgot or the school form you didn't sign. Don't forget the magical moments where everything went right and you had everything to do with it.

//

The pressure to be everything for everyone took root deep in my core long before I even noticed, long before I became a mom. Over the course of my life, it took me over the edge and back again more times than I can count. I suffered my first panic attack during those first few months of "cohabitation" with Gani. My anxiety became so big, I started digging through my old tool box of unhealthy coping mechanisms to get by. And it wasn't until I had my daughter, my lucky star, that I had to face that anxiety head-on. I had to turn the spotlight on what it was, why it was there, and how I could finally take responsibility for it.

Chapter 10: Tally Marks

'm just reopening wounds at this point. Going over marks I've already sliced open. Dragging the metal point against my skin to draw blood. I just want to stop hurting.

It's a pain that I can control; a pain that I can anticipate. And I can just walk into any craft store, pick one up, and use it however I want. There's no warning on the box. *Don't operate X-Acto knife during depressive episodes. Don't use it to slice the inside of your arm. Don't drag it across your skin until you see blood.*

It's a relief. I sit on the floor of my bathroom and find sweet relief. Most people find relief in the bathroom in other ways. I come here to find protection. To feel safe.

My relief comes as I sit with my back hunched against the side of the tub, my head leaning back over the ledge letting the tears roll themselves out of my eyes, down my cheeks, and into my ears. I sit there, totally still, ears filling with tears like my head is submerged underwater. Like drowning.

I curl into the fetal position next to the toilet and make myself as small as I can.

//

The scratches on my arms became tally marks. Every time I would get triggered, my immediate reaction was to run away from the feelings that came with that trigger. And so, I'd grab the sharpest object I could find, and I'd run to the bathroom. I'd scratch line after line into my arm until the feeling passed. They were tally marks.

Maybe I was counting down to something. How many times can I do this? How many times is too much? They also served as physical proof. Something was hurting me and I couldn't prove it. But these marks, the faint red lines scabbing over the skin on the inside of my forearm, they proved it. This is how many times I have been hurt. This is how many times I have felt a pain I couldn't understand or explain. *This* is how many times.

//

The first time I cut myself, I was pregnant with my daughter. I had never cut myself before, but I had been doing plenty of self-harm up until that point. I was unconsciously self-medicating and developing unhealthy coping mechanisms to solve a problem I didn't really know I had: anonymous sex, binge drinking, excessive dieting, and mindless scrolling, to name a few. Anything to drown out the noise, numb the pain, and feel like I was in control.

I used to make myself throw up. There are many more layers to that story, but those are the bare bones of it. I used to make myself throw up and I had a hard time finding a name for it. And it wasn't until I began finding a name for it that I truly began to overcome it.

Bulimia is defined as a serious eating disorder marked by binging, followed by methods to avoid weight gain. I'll admit I've had a complicated relationship with food and suffered many years of poor body image. And I will say that my eating has been disordered in the past, where I often ate to satisfy emotions rather than hunger. So, it seems natural to categorize this behavior as an eating disorder. But the better acquainted I became with my purging, the more I understood it was never about eating.

It had little to do with eating, or my body, or controlling my consumption, and had everything to do with ridding myself of certain emotions— anxiety, stress, sadness, grief. If I was overwhelmed with any one of these emotions, or sometimes all of them at once, I just wanted to press the eject button and push them out. Erase them with the flick of a finger.

I haven't acted on the impulse in a few years, mainly because I began to understand this was not something for me to just recover from, it was something for me to overcome. Because the impulse is just my immediate reaction—I may not always be able to stop it from popping into my head, but I could overcome it when it shows up.

There are still times I want to reach my finger down my throat and pull out whatever is upsetting me. I want to curl my finger around it and pull it up through my throat and out of my mouth. I crave the release. But the better I got at denying the impulse, the less immediate of a reaction it became. I dedicated myself to developing healthier reactions to stress and they soon took its place.

Sometimes the impulse is relentless. The pressure rising up my throat, poking at the back of my tongue daring me to release it. But I don't. Because I made that promise to myself. I promised myself to stop. I didn't promise my parents, or my husband, or my therapist. I made that promise to myself and only I could hold myself accountable.

I promised to never make an excuse or justify it like I had in the past. No, I wasn't drunk. No, I didn't overeat. No, that food wasn't expired. My stomach wasn't upset. I didn't need to throw up. I wanted to. That's the distinction.

I wanted to throw up. I wanted to because I liked how it felt. I liked the ritual of it. I liked the feeling of release. I liked feeling empty and hollow, scraping my insides clean of any negative emotion that was clinging to my sides, hiding under my ribs. But rather than do that, I write this. I share my story and talk about it, make it a conversation. Because the sooner we talk about it, the sooner it loses its power.

My biggest challenge in overcoming this obstacle came when I got food poisoning. Already a violent experience in itself, it was only made worse when I tried to stop myself from getting sick. I had convinced myself I would never throw up again and got angry for feeling like I needed to. I couldn't distinguish whether I was actually sick or making it up. Did I need to or want to? My body and mind were disconnected.

This visceral experience taught me a valuable lesson. We must listen to our bodies. They know so much more than we do.

Rather than deny the impulse in an attempt to overcome it, I now practice reflecting on the reckless feeling and recognizing it for what it really is: a defense mechanism. I used my purging as a way to not feel what I'm afraid to feel and as a barrier attempting to protect my heart from negative emotions. When the truth is, we don't need protection from negative emotions. We need to welcome them with open arms. Feel them, become intimate with them, know them by name. It is then that we can truly appreciate all the good things we have.

Defense mechanisms come in all shapes and forms and destructive habits. But all they are are mental blocks, emotional walls, that lock the good out and keep the bad in. When we knock them down we can finally see from a more positive perspective and let the good into our lives. The longer we fight to keep them up, the longer those negative emotions will continue stirring inside of us, finding any way they can to break out.

Like I said, I consider dealing with my binging and purging impulse as a matter of overcoming, not recovering. Putting it into those terms for myself gave me the perspective I needed to take it seriously. Someone else's experience is certainly going to be different. But the solution has to be the same: to stop. Purging is not sustainable. It began to ravage my immune system, mental health, and slowly but surely, my teeth. I was constantly tired and getting sick so easily I was in and out of Urgent Care more times than I can count. All because I was stripping my body of the nutrients it needed to sustain itself. As soon as I started to call it what it was, I began to reclaim control. The more honestly I discuss it with those around me, the weaker it becomes. The stigma disappears along with the shame and the guilt.

You see, self-destructive impulses and compulsions have a way of disguising themselves. In rituals, in superstitions, in comforts. And everyone has at least one. Some are inconveniences while others are life-threatening. I urge everyone to reflect honestly about these behaviors to determine if you should seek help. If you see that your behavior is affecting your health, your relationships, or your identity, it's time to start calling it for what it is and helping yourself overcome it.

//

Binging and purging have always been my go-to coping mechanisms. In the literal sense, of course. Binging on food and purging it back up. But I'd also binge-drink to black out, purging in the morning, hungover and regretful. I'd binge-date and quickly put out to feel loved, then purge all men from my life, vowing never to date again. My personality is very all-or-nothing.

But those prescriptions didn't work when I got pregnant. I couldn't throw up because it might hurt the baby. I couldn't binge-drink. I couldn't have anonymous sex with some stranger.

But the compulsion was still there. I was still absolutely ridden with anxiety and needed a quick fix. Therapy and recovery aren't quick. So when the compulsion would strike, maybe after an intense argument with my husband, I'd dig my nails deep into the skin of my arm until the skin broke. I'd drag my finger back and forth, digging a trench into my skin. And when that stopped scratching the itch, I graduated to using the X-Acto knife.

I wasn't suicidal. I didn't want to die. But, I was having intrusive suicidal thoughts. I've since learned this is called Suicidal OCD. Suicidal OCD is a subtype of OCD in which people fear they will lose control and kill themselves. For example, I've sat with the knife to my arm thinking, *What if I just cut deeper this time. What would happen?* I've asked my husband to hide his sleeping pills, telling him I didn't want the kids to find them, but really, I didn't want to know where they were. Because once, during a particular dark spell, I had the idea of just taking them all.

I never wanted to die, but I did want evidence that I was in pain. I wanted proof.

I just needed to distract myself from the pain I was feeling, the pain I didn't want to confront. So I'd replace it with a pain I could control. I'd take the tip of the X-Acto knife and scratch it into the skin on the inside of my arm. Back and forth, back and forth. It was almost meditative. Like watching the waves crash up onto the shore, retreat, and be brought back again. I'd calm down from whatever episodic meltdown I was in the middle of. I'd find my center at the tip of that blade.

And then, as I sat there shattered on the bathroom floor, I'd look at the fresh scratches on my arm and feel an overwhelming sense of guilt. *How could I be doing this to my body? My body is carrying life. The life of my perfect daughter. I need to stop. I will stop.*

I gave myself this pep talk plenty of times, but always ended up coming back to the knife. Until one day I decided to divulge my secret to my husband. Speak it out loud. And as soon as I admitted to him what I was doing, I finally felt a real responsibility to quit. I felt accountable. I felt supported. So I asked him to walk to our bathroom with me. I showed him where I stashed the blade. I asked him to come with me to the kitchen and watch me throw it out in the garbage. It was harder to let go of than I was expecting. But knowing that he saw me dispose of it made me that much more accountable to stop.

I gave myself a few more scratches after that, I'll be honest. My anxiety wasn't suddenly cured and I still felt the urge and often acted on it. I'd use my fingernails or bite the rubber off the end of a bobby pin. But eventually, slowly, I stopped. I stopped for her.

And whenever I look down at the faint white scars on my arm, I see her. I'm reminded that I need to be stronger, for her. I need to take responsibility of my mental health, for her. I need to be an example, for her. My daughter, my star, my little voice. Up until having her, I was simply surviving with my anxiety. It wasn't until becoming her mother and staring down into the swirling universe that lives in her eyes that I realized I could thrive with anxiety.

These are hard things to share. But sharing them relinquishes their control. As soon as I learned this, I started to use my social media accounts as a healing tool. Sharing this side of life, life on the other side of the filters, let me take control over the dark and heavy things that weigh me down. I found the more I shared, the more I served my online community. The posts that get the most engagement and garner the most connection, without fail, are the ones that are the hardest for me to hit publish on. And when I started realizing that, my relationship with social media became the healthiest it's ever been.

Stories connect us. Connection heals us. And healing lets us grow.

Chapter II: We Must Break To Let The Light In

One night, I cracked. I cracked open and fell to the floor in a million pieces. Scattered. Messy. Broken.

Eight months postpartum and my anxiety suddenly lurked back into my chest. Of course, there were blaring, blatant warnings. I just did what I always do with those warnings and ignored them.

I don't have time to deal with it, I thought.

It'll go away on its own, I thought.

I'm stronger than my anxiety, I thought.

I thought wrong.

That night my arms finally gave out. I couldn't hold the weight anymore. My knees buckled. And I cracked. I hadn't experienced a panic attack like that in a few years. It doubled me over. The pain so physical, yet so impossible to explain.

The next morning, I woke up and promised myself to start fresh. A new day. And as I wrote in my journal, the healing words flooded out of me. And I took care of myself the best way I know how: writing. I let go and let the words flow out of me from a place I often forget to tap into. A place deep in my belly where I know all the answers really are but I'm too scared or lazy or stubborn to look for them.

And I wrote the words I needed to hear. I wrote that it's okay to crack because that's how the light gets in. I wrote that my focus needs to be forward. I wrote that now is the time to clear and clean and cleanse. I wrote that I'm going to be okay. I promised myself. I'm going to be okay.

Have you ever heard of *kintsugi*? It is the Japanese art of repairing broken pottery with gold. As a philosophy, it treats breakage and repair as part of the history of an object, rather than something to disguise. I've decided to treat my repair the same way.

//

It wasn't until after giving birth to my daughter and realizing I was suffering from postpartum anxiety that I understood anxiety is something I've been dealing with my entire life. Sure, I'd seen some therapists, and they'd used the word anxiety plenty of times, but it never stuck. Not until holding her in my arms and knowing that she was looking at me to teach her and guide her, did I finally take ownership of my mental health. It is MY responsibility to get better. And in my recovery process I discovered a few things I'd been doing to self-sabotage. I noticed some things I'd been using as crutches to cope with my anxiety that really only served to make it worse.

A coping mechanism is an adaptation to environmental stress that is based on conscious or unconscious choice and that enhances control over behavior or gives psychological comfort. The key word here being *control.* You see, we think we have a lot more control over things than we actually do. So, these coping mechanisms are really only tricking us into believing we're controlling our environment or our experience, when in reality we're just running from it.

Some coping mechanisms are harmful and self-destructive. For example, making yourself throw up as a way to escape negative emotions. Even though it took me some time to finally stop, I generally knew the entire time that what I was doing was bad for me. However, some self-destructive coping mechanisms *aren't* so obvious.

Nothing will make you feel less in control than having a newborn. So while I was learning to deal with my postpartum anxiety, mechanisms I was using to feel like I was in control became obvious to me in a way they hadn't before. These coping mechanisms, which I've had in some way or another my whole life, are directly related to how anxious I feel on a daily basis.

The first is my need for order. When I break it down like that, getting all the way to the root, it's very clear that my "need for order" is a direct response to my anxiety, which flares up whenever I'm forced to experience any disorder. But, on the surface, it's not as obvious.

I always just thought I was an organized person. I like things to be in their place. I like having everything neat and clean and orderly. And when things aren't that way, I become anxious, overwhelmed, and like I'll never be able to get everything cleaned up. And so I become more overwhelmed. And I lose all motivation. And start feeling like I'm a total failure. Because if I can't do the dishes, I might as well not do anything.

You can see where my problem is. In tricking myself into believing that I can control my environment by keeping everything in order, I'm setting myself up for failure when things inevitably become disorderly. I live with four other people, three of them children, a giant dog, and a very furry cat. My house rarely looks perfect. And it shouldn't have to! We *live* here.

The other coping mechanism I've discovered is my need for routine. As long as everything is the same and nothing changes, I'm not anxious. Again, saying it like this, it sounds very obvious what my problem is. However, day to day, I wasn't able to see it.

All I was able to notice was that when my routine would falter even just the slightest bit, my entire day would be ruined. If plans changed. If I had to step a single foot outside of my comfort zone. Any change at all would cause me to seize up. But, just like disorder is a constant in life, so is change. Both things are inevitable and very much out of our control.

A third coping mechanism I discovered was depression. I don't mean to say I consciously employed this very serious disease in order to run from my problems. But, I do believe my mind went there as a way to cope with the chaos and disorder that was triggering my anxiety.

My on-again, off-again relationship with depression came in tandem with my on-again, off-again relationship with social media. I didn't put those pieces together at the time, but now I understand just how revealing that is.

Chapter 12: Trigger Warning

The internet has become bad for my health, so I'll be taking a break from social media until further notice.

In the few weeks after returning from our wedding and honeymoon, I fell into a depression. Some might think that's normal to experience after a wedding. Especially one as perfect as ours was. But, that is not what triggered it.

This is what triggered it.

I used to go to the gym at the local JCC. That stands for Jewish Community Center. My stepsons went to daycare, preschool, and summer camp there. It's a pillar in our community and I'm happy to have been a member.

After the gym, I would go into the sauna after I worked out so I could look more sweaty. I had made it my goal to use that time to meditate. One day, as I sat in the sauna, I had gotten through about a minute and a half of an audio recording of mantra meditation before I started to get antsy. I had this nervous feeling demanding my attention. That's normal while meditating, but I couldn't move past it like I usually do. So, frustrated with myself, I took out my earphones and headed out.

As I walked out of the locker room, I saw a mass of people exiting all at once. I assumed it was just an exercise class being let out. But then I noticed a panic on everyone's faces, and I realized it wasn't just some people leaving the gym…it was all the people running out the door. So, I stopped a woman and asked what was going on. She told me a bomb threat had been called in and everyone was being evacuated.

Before going to the gym, I had dropped my youngest step son off at the preschool next door. Upon hearing of the bomb threat, I ran to his class only to find the doors locked. No one in, no one out. So

I, along with a few other moms, waited there in front of the door like sitting ducks. No one knew what was going on or how serious or imminent the threat was. Eventually, an administrator opened the door, saying, "We don't know what's going on, but you can go get your kids and run." So, I did. I ran down the hall, scooped him up in my arms, and ran back to my car, still not knowing if or when something might happen. I sped home, picking up his older brother from the nearby public school on the way, just in case. I told them school was closed for early release, and they were happy to stay home. I spent the day refreshing my News Feeds, desperate to learn more, but almost no one was talking about it. It ended up being a hoax phone call, just like the other hundreds around the country.

Then, the following Tuesday, it happened again. As I dropped my stepson off, another threat got called in and we were put on lockdown. They locked us in a classroom and closed all the blinds. God bless the teachers who can act in moments like these. They let me out and I made a run for it, getting out the door with him to my car just before complete campus lockdown. Again, the "all clear" was announced hours later and normal activities resumed. Another hoax phone call.

Of course, before these events, I had already been consuming all the scary news stories and feeling all the fear that type of content was intended to incite. But I still never thought it would touch me. Then it did. And all I could think was, if I'm feeling this scared right now in my safe upper-class white suburban neighborhood, with its gated communities and private schools and choice of organic food stores and yoga studios, how is everyone else feeling? Everyone else who isn't safe and privileged like I am.

So, to recap.

Here I am, simultaneously reading about the active rewind of our nation's progress, while grieving for all the lives that are being touched by it, while feeling privileged for not being touched by it, while envying the beautiful and perfect lives of the people I follow online, while living my own beautiful and perfect life, while experiencing two bomb threats back-to-back.

It just didn't add up. And my brain, it seems, short-circuited in its effort to try and make sense of it all. That short-circuiting manifested as depression.

At this point, I still had a lot to sort-out regarding my depression. But, what I did know was that this time I could recognize it and identify it a lot sooner. I found myself incapacitated, sucked dry of any motivation. All I could bring myself to do was sit on the couch. And when I wasn't staring blankly out the window, I was scrolling through my phone. Hours spent arbitrarily consuming content, both terrifying and glamorous. I just kept feeling more sick and more isolated the more content I consumed.

Eventually, I recognized that it wasn't making me feel good. I couldn't place it, but I just knew that scrolling through my phone wasn't helping. In fact, it was doing the exact opposite. So, I signed off in an effort to try and feel better. And during that time, I made some pretty powerful assessments that I'd like to share with you.

I had found myself dangling between two starkly contrasting realities that I was attempting to participate in. The one I wished was fake (current state of affairs) and the one I knew to be fake (social media). But neither of them are real. Neither of them have anything to do with me and my life and my experience and my existence.

And then I realized, I hadn't been participating in my own existence as a person here on earth and instead had traded it in to play a part in these elaborate alternate realities.

What the fuck?

And then I started thinking, I can't be the only one doing this. We must be all doing this, collectively. And, with that thought, we must all be collectively really fucking depressed.

Because the contrast between real life and online portrayals of life has become despairingly divided. So much so that it's becoming almost impossible to have a relationship with either one. The contrast is so confounded, we are all stuck in the space between the two deciding which one to reach toward. The one we wish was fake or the one we know is fake.

And while we're debating over the two, real life is happening without us. Like, real life. Our life. Day-to-day life. And that is a damn shame. And a waste of time.

Okay, thanks for bumming us all out. But now what!

Imagine what we could be doing with that time! We've become too comfortable existing within that contrast. We need to take back our time and decide for ourselves how we want to spend it, because right now we're spending our time arguing about which is the right way instead of finding our own way.

So, that's what I intend to do, and what I encourage you to do. Let's each find our own way.

I recognized then that I needed to find my own equilibrium between that which is me and that which is outside of me, between that which I can control and that which I can't. We can't achieve a collective balance until we each individually achieve our own. And that takes making a concerted, intentional effort.

Chapter 13: The Comparison Game

We all get caught up in it. We find ourselves envying the lives others are pretending to live online. We start desiring something, and working toward something, that doesn't even exist. And what's worse, we start to discredit and remove ourselves from the miraculous reality we're already a part of. We need to learn how to avoid the comparison game online.

The tricky thing about this game is that we all know it's fake, yet it somehow continues to trick us. We know that what we're posting isn't what our life looks like in its entirety, and yet it's so hard to remember that that's true for everyone else who is posting and sharing pieces of their lives online.

The truth is, what we're doing is filtering our realities. Each of us is doing this. We are taking our real lives and presenting them online with a veil of perfection. Because why not? I'd much rather show a picture of me smiling on vacation than me crying in the shower because I'm PMS-ing. Both are equally real parts of my life. But one I'm excited to share with the world, while the other I'd prefer keeping to myself (plus no one really wants to see that.)

The thing to remember is that behind each of those veils of perfection is real life. Each of us has our own multifaceted, confusing, thrilling, happy, exhausting, miserable, beautiful REAL life. With crying babies and messy kitchens and boring weekends and cellulite.

So, how then do we navigate this online landscape and show up to do our work without constantly getting derailed by the comparison game? How do we use the internet and social media while taking full advantage of all their resources in order to reach the people who need us? How do we create content that works online without falling into the trap of manipulating our actual realities in an attempt to look like what we're seeing works online?

We need to separate the reality we share online from the reality we live offline.

And the best way I've learned to do this is by setting boundaries, or mental reminders, to keep myself from falling down the rabbit hole that is the online comparison game.

//

My husband has teenaged nieces and nephews. I was speaking to his niece once, I think she was sixteen at the time. There was only one tiny decade sitting between her and I, but the faster technology is advancing, the faster that gap between generations is becoming an ever-expanding chasm. To her, social media is just another extension of her existence. It's not a tool so much as it's another mode of communication. Like AOL Instant Messenger once was to me.

That day, she explained to me that she had a fake Instagram account to share pictures with her real friends. Yeah, it didn't make sense to me either. But she let me know that this is actually quite common. It's called a "Finstagram," for all you other old biddies out there scratching your heads. Basically, she has a separate account where she posts pictures of herself doing normal sixteen-year-old things like making silly faces and having sleepovers and being in high school.

What, then, does her "real" Instagram account feature? Well, for one thing, thousands of followers. But also buzzworthy pictures of her doing more exciting things like attending concerts and going out on boats and wearing trendy clothes with her friends. You see, those things are still a part of her reality. They might not represent her day-to-day, or the majority of what she does with her time. But they're the pretty, perfect, shiny, exciting highlight reel. So why not share them?

One thing I think we can take away from all this is her firm understanding of the separation between her actual reality and the one she shares online. When she explained her "fake" account with her real friends, she did so with such matter-of-factness. She knew exactly what she was doing online and had a firm boundary in place. Is it time-consuming? Sure. Is she still doing things just for the sake of taking pictures? Maybe. But, our generation will never fully understand or relate to the ones who come after us and we shouldn't try. They know something we don't, just like we knew something our parents didn't.

This is at least what I hope to be true. In my gut, though, I still fear for the generation following us. I fear that they might be so consumed with turning their life into likable content that they're missing out on just being kids while they can. But what do I know? I'm ancient!

I want to encourage all of us, myself included, to know the difference when we're sharing our lives online. Let us post our content knowing that we're posting the highlight reel. This will help create that instinctual boundary. For her, social media is primarily another form of communication, like the telephone once was to talking.

For a lot of us, social media serves as a platform to get in front of people who need our services or to make money for ourselves and our families through paid sponsorships. For the rest of us, it's simply a place to keep in touch with our friends and families, much like when we used to send holiday cards. Maybe the big shift is just treating your News Feed like an infinitely-scrolling, constantly-updating holiday card.

//

Comparison is the thief of joy.
This whole social media mindfuck is so much deeper than any of us realize. We are so rooted in this online existence, we don't see where our real selves start and our online personas end. We've grown up online. I can at least remember a time before I had a Facebook. I'm one of the lucky ones. Social media didn't fall into my lap until I was graduating high school. And even then, it was nothing like it is today. We didn't use it the same way. We were just playing around with a new toy, blissfully unaware of its staying power. Unaware of how it was morphing us, as a species.

I believe that the advent of social media has sparked the next phase of evolution for our species. Think about it. Up until now, our brains never had to perform like this. We had a finite amount of people that we interacted with on a daily basis. We could only compare ourselves to those physically around us. Maybe we saw actresses and models in magazine ads and on the screen, but there was an understood distance there. We merely had to look around our physical space to gauge our expectations. Maybe there was that one cool girl in class with all the trendy clothes that everyone wanted to be. Or that one perfect mom who made it to every school event and baked the cookies and always looked put-together. We'd see them. We'd romanticize their life. But it wouldn't go much further.

Now? It's such a different story. It's a story that's never been told. Now all I need to do is open up an app on my phone to see millions of cool girls in trendy clothes and millions of perfect moms who seemingly have it all together. I can read millions of articles telling me to live life one way followed by another million telling me to do the exact opposite. Our brains are not cut out for this type of mental gymnastics. We haven't been programmed to sift through this amount of noise.

And we're suffering. Rates of depression, anxiety, and suicide are higher than they've ever been. Especially amongst teenagers. We're willingly giving up our freedom. Our anonymity. Our privacy. For what? For likes and follows? For the dream of "going viral?" For fame? What is it? What is driving us to stay in this system? Why can't we unplug and opt out?

I'm not sure. I ask myself this question constantly. Constantly deleting the apps off my phone only to redownload them the next day. Deactivating my Facebook only to miss seeing what all of my friends are up to. I hate being online, but I can't stay away.

So the question becomes, how can we help our brains evolve to exist harmoniously within this new system? How can we train our brains to clearly see the distinction between real life and online life? Because up until now, we've made no effort to create that distinction. Right now, they're one in the same.

The answer, I'm learning, is boundaries.

The other day I caught myself filming my daughter and was struck by this overwhelming feeling that we're in trouble. I caught her doing something funny and pulled out my camera to film her.

And I realized as I was filming her that I was watching the moment through my phone. Rather than watching her play with her toys and babble to herself, I was watching her on my phone screen as I was recording it. And a wave of nausea washed over me. Because it felt like when I mindlessly tap through Instagram stories and consume videos of other people's kids, voyeuristically watching their lives online. I was doing the same with my own life, with my own kid. What the fuck is that? That's fucked up. I felt sick.

It's as if my entire life is just potential content waiting to be staged and filtered and posted. Like my real life is just the prop room backstage.

We're doing this whole thing backwards. We're living these fabricated lives online and treating our real lives as fodder. We should be going online to learn things. To ask questions. Find answers. Connect. But we aren't. We're going online and…living. It's like we sign into Instagram and suddenly we're in this giant high school auditorium comparing ourselves to everyone else around us. There's no time to connect when all we can do is compare. And I'm not sure we're going to turn that impulse off. So what's the solution?

We can't just unplug. We're living here already. We're settled in. And we can't just close our eyes and not look at everyone else living here and not compare ourselves to them. So what? How can we continue doing this without going insane?

I don't know.

One thing I feel like I really need to do is get back in touch with what's real. Integrate back into the real world. The physical world. Where I can only compare myself to the moms I meet in person. Where I'm only seeing their kids in person, as they play with my kids. Where I dress myself up because I like how it makes me feel, I cook a beautiful meal because it's fun, and I capture a brilliant sunset because I want to remember it forever.

//

When I became pregnant with my daughter, I completely abandoned social media. I had been having a rocky relationship with it up until then and becoming pregnant pushed me over the edge. It wasn't until about twenty-six weeks in that I started to feel the itch to come back. Why? Because I wanted to share with my friends and family. I liked keeping up with my loved ones. However, I was also keeping up with the Kardashians. And the Real Housewives. And every other stranger I was following around on the internet.

That's when I decided that if I were to come back online, I was going to do it my way. I begrudgingly came to the conclusion that Facebook was the most convenient way for me to stay in touch with friends and family. It was impractical for me to send individual texts and emails to everyone I love when I wanted to share some news or stay up-to-date on their lives.

So, I did what I could, whittling down my friends list to only include those who I actually know and love. Maybe it was a part of that third trimester nesting bug, but I was decluttering every nook and cranny of my life...including my Facebook.

I still kept my social media engagement fairly sparse, but I couldn't help but want to share this next chapter with friends and family. I made my pages private. I meticulously selected who sees my posts. I tried to be as conscious as I could be about who I was choosing to share my life with and how. That's what irked me so much to begin with and drove me from the platform entirely. Everyone doesn't need to know everything I'm doing. But my close friends and family who care to know, should. And I've found this is the easiest means of doing that.

I'm conscious about who is consuming my content and conscious about what content I am consuming. I unfollow accounts without abandon, I block users I don't feel comfortable with, I privatize my personal accounts and pick and choose what parts of my personal life to share on my public ones. I'm slowly regaining control of how I use this thing.

I've taken more breaks than Ross and Rachel, but I finally feel like I've found my balance with social media. I have been figuring out how to make a space for myself online that isn't a mindless, soul-sucking cesspool.

Really consider: Why do you post what you post? Why do you follow the accounts that you follow? Are they friends you want to keep in touch with? Are they strangers who offer inspiration? Do they make you laugh, think, feel? Or have you not really put too much thought into at all?

I ran a poll on my Instagram stories once in an effort to better understand my audience, asking them about their social media consumption habits. If I'm going to be online, I want to add value to their lives and create content they want to consume. However, I learned that most people don't really know what content they want to consume. They just consume it, mindlessly scrolling out of boredom.

That's the trap. By the time we swipe our thumb up on our screen, blindly find the Instagram app, tap it open and start scrolling, we've already been sucked in without realizing it. We don't even know how we got there.

I think this is just one of the downfalls of the social media machine and a big reason we all feel not so great about using it. We still use it, of course. Whether you're using it to make money through paid sponsorships, build an audience platform to sell your next book, or just use it to stay in touch with friends and family, it's not realistic to be off the stuff for good.

So, what can we do? How can we exist with this technology and use it in a way that adds value to our lives? My suggestion is setting boundaries, becoming conscious of how we're using these apps, and what type of content we're consuming.

Below are a few ways I've tried to set boundaries with social media use. So far, I feel like they're working. I still feel like being on social media can be a gigantic waste of time. But these tips allow me to make my time on the apps more meaningful and productive.

1. Deleting the apps off your phone

I've done this a few times. Right now I just keep the Instagram app on my phone, because I'm making a push to build a stronger platform there. Plus, I like hanging out there. But the idea is to delete the apps off your phone, even if just for a week, to see how often you find yourself flipping open your screen and looking for the apps. It's a lot more often than you realize.

Another trick I've tried is grouping all the social media apps into the same folder, moving that folder to the last screen of apps and titling it something that forces me to pay attention. Like "Bored?" or "Are you sure?" You can also try signing out every time you leave the app. That way, when you go back and it asks you to sign in, you get to pause for a moment to decide whether or not you really need to be there.

2. Unfollowing people you don't know or don't add value

We forget that we are in control of who we follow online. Over the years, in an effort to get more followers, I had followed thousands of strangers around the internet. This left me consuming the content of a bunch of strangers, and when I signed back online after being away for so long I realized I had no reason to be following most of them.

So, when I signed back online I would scroll through my Instagram feed and stop myself every time I saw an account I didn't recognize or didn't necessarily enjoy, and I'd unfollow them. In the process, I lost a ton of followers, like fifty in a week from what I remember. But, as much as I'm back online to focus on building my platform, followers who aren't consuming my content and instead only follow me because I follow them are not the audience I'm focused on growing.

Now when I go on Instagram, I enjoy myself. I see content that makes me laugh, think, feel. It motivates me to try new things. It's content I want to be consuming.

3. Privatize your private accounts

When it came to my personal accounts, I made them super private and deleted anybody who I didn't personally know and regularly interact with. Now when I post about my family and my kids, I know who is consuming that content. I know it is only people I am allowing to see it, the friends and family who care to see it.

This made me a lot more comfortable posting updates, which I had missed doing but started hating because I didn't like strangers seeing pictures of my kids and my vacations. Now I can share updates with friends and family and keep up with theirs in a way that makes more sense to me.

4. Find alternatives to relieve boredom

Finally, the best boundary to set is to find alternatives to these apps. We don't NEED to be on social media as much as we are. We go there because we're bored. We're nursing the baby for the millionth time that day. We're sitting in the waiting room. We're lying in bed at the end of the day too tired to do anything else.

But, there are alternatives: books, music, writing, painting, dancing, even stepping outside and just looking around. My favorite is podcasts! That's why I decided to start my own.

But in general, I'd say find other fun ways to use your phone. Or bring books with you when you know you're going to be waiting somewhere. Or just enjoy the moment of silence and stillness. Just sit there and be. I fear we're forgetting how to do that.

These are just a few ways I've come up with to set boundaries with social media. It's helping, to an extent. I'm starting to be more mindful of the content I'm consuming. I'm trying to be more conscious about the content I am creating. If we're going to be here anyway, I want to at least make it a place that adds value to our lives. Not insecurity, judgment, self-doubt, loneliness, and seething rage.

Chapter 14: Freedom

I t's 2001 and I'm sitting in my sixth-grade science classroom, first period. I turn to my desk mate, Alexandra, to ask to borrow one of her glitter rainbow gel pens. As the teacher is scribbling the day's assignment onto the chalkboard at the front of the room, Alexandra and I proceed to draw intricate swirls and doodle hearts up and down our arms. The room is full of innocent, pre-pubescent eleven-year-olds, whispering to one another about music lyrics and cartoons and sports teams.

My friends and I were in the gifted program in middle school. It was called "Global Academy." This meant we all had the same group of teachers. Our science teacher, Mrs. Stanley, was a small, thin-framed Jewish woman from New York. Our English teacher, Mrs. Nichols, was an angry old broad who despised when we'd click our pens in class. Our math teacher, Mrs. Gay, would give us full-sized Nerds Rope candy for answering particularly hard problems. Our entire group was very close-knit and somewhat isolated from the rest of the school.

On this morning, as my arms were covered in glitter gel ink, Mrs. Nichols stormed through the door of our classroom and ran up to Mrs. Stanley in what seemed like a panic. We couldn't make out what she was saying, but both women seemed visibly shaken and the entire energy in the room suddenly became very tense and anxious, as if we all collectively began holding our breath.

Before we knew it, Mrs. Stanley had turned the TV on. Neither woman said anything to the confused group of eleven-year-olds darting fearful stares back and forth at each other over their Bunsen burners.

The screen turned on and we saw a skyscraper that was on fire. Was it on fire? Wait, what did they say? A plane?

And before we could piece together what the news anchor's voice was saying behind the image on our screen, we all sat there and watched as United Airlines Flight 175 flew into the World Trade Center.

We were a classroom of eleven-year-old children, most of whom didn't even know what the World Trade Center was. Children. We were children and we watched an airplane full of people fly into a giant skyscraper full of even more people. On live television.

This is the moment that separates my generation from those before us and those after us. Those of us who were children on September 11, 2001. Our entire lives were effectively shaped by this one catastrophic moment. Sure, we'd seen others. The Columbine High School massacre from a few years before, and its subsequent news coverage, made us scared to go to school. We all watched, too young to understand, as our sitting president got on television and declared he "did not have sexual relations with that woman." That entire classroom of eleven-year-olds lived through Hurricane Andrew for crying out loud, with most of our homes in the direct eye. We'd seen some shit.

But this. This was bigger than all of it. That day shifted our entire world on its axis. A tidal wave of fear rushed over our country overnight. Words we'd never heard before—like insurgents, extremists, Muslims, and terrorists—were being plastered on every TV screen.

We were too young to make sense of it, of course, but it left a permanent imprint on our collective psyche. A seed was planted that day into the consciousness of my generation. A seed of fear that would grow into an invasive plant in our minds, fruiting mental illness and hate and racism and phobias. Just as we were about to open our eyes and understand the world around us, the world around us became a place where airplanes fly into buildings on American soil. That is our normal. We saw it with our own eyes. Of course we'd be certain it would happen again. Of course we'd be scared of "terrorists". Of course we'd believe what the media told us. To be a child during that time, watching that plane fly into that building in real time, it primed us to be forever fearful. Of our surroundings, of the unknown, of "others."

Just like my classmates and I were isolated from the rest of the school, confined in the bubble of our gifted program, so, too, is our entire generation. We have come of age within this bubble of constant news coverage, viral media, and fear tactics. It's not that life is getting worse and scarier per se, we're just able to see more of the bad and scary parts of life than we ever were able to before the internet. That's just our normal. We're used to reading terrifying headlines and watching shiny news reporters tell us what to be scared of. We grew up with this. And now that we're adults, we're desperate for an escape

So where do we go? We go online. To the filtered photos and silly cat videos and infinite scrolls and "If you were a sandwich, which would you be?" questionnaires. It's become our escape. But it's also where they feed us more fear, through their weaponized media and viral news stories. Their algorithms and their data-mining. It is a vicious cycle.

I think it's time to break that cycle. And I think we're just the ones to do it.

//

Recovering from anxiety is realizing the only thing you can control in this life is yourself: what you think, what you feel, how you react, who you choose to surround yourself with, what you eat, what you buy, how you pray.

What I found to be the biggest thing standing in the way between me and my recovery was social media. The internet. The screens telling me how to live my life. The thing taking control over the only thing I'll ever have control over: my mind. If anxiety is fear of losing control, it is no surprise we are all so anxious. So fearful. Afraid of getting it wrong. Afraid of missing out. Afraid we are failing. Paranoia.

This mind-fucking has been going on for generations, don't be mistaken. I just think our generation is experiencing it in a more condensed, constant, subconscious way than any generation before us. We are not the first to be tricked into buying shit we don't need. We are not the first to fund corrupt industries and look the other way because we're willfully ignoring the truth. Because the buzzy pictures and loud talking heads on the screens are really good at their jobs. They're really good at blowing that smoke and hanging up those mirrors.

And I was one of the people coming up with ways to trick you into buying those things. Hi, I'm Lauren. And I used to work late coming up with advertising campaigns to convince mothers to give their babies sugar water. I used to glamorize the healthcare industry and sell doctors and medicine to the highest bidder. I was an account executive at a creative advertising agency. And I'm sorry.

//

Have you ever heard the term "torches of freedom?" It might conjure up Lady Liberty perched atop her platform, waving her flaming torch at hopeful immigrants as they made their way to Ellis Island. Or of runners all over the world passing off a fiery torch one-by-one as it makes its way to the Olympic Game's opening ceremony. Celebration. Hope. Honor. Freedom.

What about tar, nicotine, chemicals, and tobacco tightly-packed and rolled into a paper tube, then lit at the end to fill the air and lungs with carcinogens and disease? Cigarettes! Torches of freedom!

When Edward Bernays, the father of modern advertising, the most successful mind-fucker we've ever seen, was given the task to sell cigarettes to women, he didn't waste any time. Why was he asked to sell cigarettes to women? Well, because the tobacco industry felt like they were missing profits from half the population and that needed to be fixed ASAP. So they called on Bernays to solve their problem. And he concocted the brilliant plan to hire women to march while smoking their "torches of freedom" in the Easter Sunday Parade of 1929.

Why? Because marching these defiant and sassy flapper girls through the streets with their "torches of freedom" was a surefire way to encourage women's smoking by exploiting their aspirations for a better life during the women's liberation movement in the United States.

Cigarettes were described as symbols of emancipation and equality with men. The term "torches of freedom" was first used by psychoanalyst A. A. Brill when describing the natural desire for women to smoke and was then used by Edward Bernays to encourage women to smoke in public despite social taboos.

I read about this successful advertising campaign in college, where I took classes to learn how to recreate it. I worked my ass off in high school to get accepted into college to spend four years learning how to sell shit to people. I learned how to package food to make it seem more appetizing, what words to use to make you feel certain emotions, where to place certain products in the store so that you're more willing to make that impulse buy. None of it is an accident. And almost none of it is up to you.

Yes, you're the consumer. And, in theory, the law of supply and demand would mean you'd get to dictate what we (the advertisers and companies that hire them) sell to you and how. You'd tell us what you want and we'd make it and sell it. However, we all know that's not how it really works, right? You DO know that we're all being told what to buy, how to dress, who to date, where to travel, who to vote for...the list is endless.

And ever since that twenty-four-hour news cycle got put into tiny screens in our hands, we have been turned into horses with feeding bags under our chins, eating it all up. As soon as we start to notice that the feedbag is there, whinnying and cocking our heads around to shake it loose, we get prodded with another jolt of electricity to get us back in line. Another bird flu, another celebrity scandal, another missing child, another mass shooting. We rediscover the bag all over again and keep our faces buried so deep we can't even see the blinders they've slid onto either side of our heads. We are the livestock. We are not in control. We are not calling the shots.

Is it any surprise, then, that we're so anxious, depressed, and dissatisfied? Why rates of suicide have increased nearly thirty percent in the past twenty years? Why we're so divided as a nation? We're being turned against each other so that we point our fingers everywhere else except where the blame actually lies. I promise that I'm not going to put on my tin foil hat and start spewing conspiracy theories of lizard king overlords or how we're living in the matrix. But I will say this: think about it. Who is winning here? Who is winning in this game? It's clearly not us. So if not us, who?

And it doesn't even really matter who, does it? I don't think so. I think what matters most here, what I want the take-away to be, is that we GET to be in control. We get to have a say: over our lives, our bodies, our wallets, our choices. And it's about time we start.

I think that starts with taking responsibility for our own mental health and how we use the internet. It is our responsibility to find a way to exist harmoniously with this technology, because we're handing it over to the next generation. To our children. And I for one refuse to hand over this hotbed of neurosis and narcissism to my kids.

I worry, though, we're so preoccupied watching everyone else's lives that we might miss our chance at doing the important work of living our own. You see, we are all plagued with chronic busyness. It's an adverse side effect to the delusion we have that everyone else is doing more than we are. We're all trying to keep up with every-one else's highlight reel, stuck in a sick feedback loop that never ends. And we don't compare our own situation to everyone else's individual situations. Instead, we compare our own situation to everyone else's situation, collectively. As a whole. And our individ-ual efforts stand no chance against what everyone else is doing, all together. Sure, we just got a new job, but she's traveling the world and he just got married and they just had a baby. We're not doing any of those things! So in order to feel like we are a part of it, we wave our busy flag and join the fight so we can keep up with all the other busy bees.

But while we're all busy being busy, life is passing us by. Rela-tionships aren't being nourished, families aren't connecting, bonds aren't forming. As we're all arguing over who has the least amount of hours in their day, opportunities for better and more full lives are being wasted. We're constantly looking outward to compare our situation to everyone else's rather than focusing that attention inward, into our own families, lives, and relationships.

The truth is, we all aren't as happy as we pretend to be on the internet. For every adorably happy baby there are hours of crying tantrums and exasperation. For every dream job landed, there are hundreds of rejection letters. Every "I said yes!" picture carries with it an anxiety of what's to come.

Life isn't perfect. For anyone. But in-between all those messy and trying moments, there is a glimmer of perfection. It just takes effort to see it. So instead of putting that effort into the excuses for why we just can't, let's put that energy into finding those glimmers of perfection. And savoring them. Not taking their picture. Not posting about them. Not chasing them. Let us witness and immerse ourselves in life. Because sometimes, it's pretty perfect.

Chapter 15: Let Go or Be Dragged

earning to put boundaries in place has led me to have a much healthier relationship with social media. I actually enjoy showing up online now. I look forward to interacting with people, reading their comments, engaging. And all I had to do was set boundaries.

BUT. And this is a big but that I don't think we talk about enough: We cannot set boundaries and hold them in place until we really sit with ourselves to learn which boundaries we need and why. We have to do the hard and tedious work of getting to know ourselves in order to figure out what boundaries we actually need. We have to understand why we need them. Only then can we put them in place and expect them to do anything.

I finally came to the conclusion that I will never be able to develop a more conscious relationship with social media until I develop a more conscious relationship with myself. My online world will never feel like a safe space until my inner world does. And that couldn't happen until I started to take responsibility for my mental health and learn how to heal from the inside, out.

//

Spirituality has always been a part of my life, even before I knew to call it that.

When I was a child I used to set up altars in my room, complete with flowers and mementos, and have conversations with my guardian angels. I would spread out an old towel and cover it with weeds from the garden that I saw as beautiful, tiny flowers. I would then find old family photos of people I never knew yet somehow felt deeply connected to, and I would kneel in front of this little make-shift shrine and speak to them. I was a child, maybe five or six years old, so these conversations were never too complex. But I'd ask how they were doing, who else was there with them, and if they could please continue watching over me and my family. I also used to tell my mom about seeing and hearing people in empty houses.

When I was in high school, my English teacher introduced me to the teachings of Buddhism. He held a meditation club after school where he taught us the principles of mindfulness and different meditation techniques. While my friends were practicing oboe or starting a girls lacrosse team, I was sitting at a desk after school learning how to breathe: How to breathe in a bright, white light, and breathe out a dark, thick smoke. How to quiet the mind, witness my thoughts, and relish in the present moment. His teachings laid the foundation for my spiritual practice.

In college I discovered yoga and took more classes on Buddhism. I read books and watched seminars and internalized the ancient teachings. After college, a friend introduced me to the Wild Unknown Tarot Deck. I had already been to a few different psychics and readers, but I had never read the cards myself. With the help of my friend, I taught myself how to read tarot, and have since incorporated it into my meditation practice, calling upon the cards when I'm in need of some reflection or insight.

Along with all of this, I also practice my spirituality from the inside out. I believe my body is a temple, and I care for it as such. Good in, good out. I've been a vegetarian for the past 10 years, choosing not to eat meat because of my sensitivity toward animals. I eat clean, natural, and organic food as often as I can. I choose to follow holistic and preventive health practices, seeing the effects and benefits of natural remedies like acupuncture. I eat bee pollen to wake up in the morning; I drink lavender tea to fall asleep. There's a collection of essential oils in my nightstand that I use to ease my anxiety, magnify my positive vibes, and promote restful sleep. More recently, I have discovered crystals and their enormous healing properties. I keep them by my bed, stuff them in my bra, and wear them around my neck and wrists.

This lifestyle can get a bad rap. I'm sure the word "spiritual" conjures up a very specific image in your head. I'm not going to illustrate it, in an effort to discontinue that stigma, but you know what I'm talking about. The words "hippy-dippy" come to mind. Or, "crunchy-granola," perhaps.

The spirituality world has become quite a scene, but don't let that keep you from its invaluable resources.

For example, I wish *everyone* did yoga. It's difficult and uncomfortable and sometimes our arms just can't twist like that! But I truly believe the practice of yoga can change lives.

The word *yoga* is derived from the Sansrkit root "yuj", which means to yoke, unite, or connect. It connects the mind, body, and soul in a way that betters our whole being. The clearer our mind is, the more open our heart can be. The leaner our muscles feel, the stronger we carry ourselves. The longer we hold that handstand, the more powerful our confidence becomes. It's all connected.

I have been practicing yoga for almost ten years now and the most important thing I've taken away is simply that we must be kind to ourselves. We can't get upset with our bodies for not performing the way they did last class, or last pose. We must love our body and relish in all it can do. Yoga practice serves as a reminder that we haven't always been able to touch our toes, or hold a warrior pose, or stand on our hands! Just as we haven't always had the courage to move to another city, or the guts to chase our dreams, or the stamina to run a mile! We are always changing, always growing. And, just as in life, sometimes we'll try and fail. But then we'll try again. And again, and again, until finally, we'll nail it! Even if just for a split second. That's all it takes to feel the epiphany. To feel ourselves open up and witness all we're capable of.

Every yoga practice is different. With each class we bring a different body. Our bones sit differently than they did last class, our muscles are tighter or looser depending on the stress we've been putting on them. But all this helps us remember to give up control. We can't force our bodies into positions they aren't ready for, just like we can't force situations to turn out the way we want them to, or force people to be something they aren't. Yoga teaches us how to give up control. It shows us how to trust the process, surrender to the universe, and know all works out as it should.

Yoga also allows for vulnerability. Bending over in tight spandex in a silent room, listening to complete strangers' labored breaths, is an intimate experience. But it builds strength and confidence and compassion. Witnessing others of all different skill levels attempt a new pose and need a few moments to become comfortable with it is a reminder that we all start from the same place. Yoga is a practice that takes time and dedication. But it brings the best reward, which is *knowing*. Knowing we are capable, knowing we are strong, knowing we can do what we once found impossible.

So I encourage everyone, regardless of age or ability, to walk into a yoga class. Walk in fearlessly, knowing you're embracing your body and inviting it to move in ways you never knew possible. Surprise yourself! And embrace the knowing that comes from within.

Sue Monk Kidd wrote in The Secret Life of Bees, "The body knows things a long time before the mind catches up to them". Yoga is about strengthening the mind-body connection. Asana, the poses we hold during practice, are like a mantra for the body. We repeat these poses over and over, holding them for long periods of time, until our bodies and minds finally reconnect.

A mantra is a phrase or sound repeated to aid concentration in meditation. Some of us may have them and not even realize we use them. I've adopted a few over the years to help ease my anxiety, re-focus my energy, and come back to my moment.

However, though they've proven themselves true time and again, I often doubt my mantras. I become fearful that I am using them as excuses. You see, I tend to over-rationalize difficult situations in an attempt to make sense of them. In my past, this has led to toxic relationships being drawn out for years and unhappy work environments being tolerated for too long. Life's uncertainty leaves me anxious about how to make the distinction between what I can and can't control.

The truth is, there is a balance that must be reached. While we must act with intention and take responsibility for our actions, we must also recognize that some circumstances in our life will be out of our control. That is a difficult thing for me to accept. And in order to make sense of it, I attempt to rationalize it, because I ache to understand the reason why things are happening. But what I'm realizing is that sometimes we won't understand that "why" until the reason is ready to present itself. So, we must practice patience. With patience we can cherish our moments, good and bad, for the lessons they are, for the steps they take us toward our future. We'll never be able to control all that life throws at us, but we will always be able to control how we react to it.

If you're anything like me, this patience can be excruciating at times. It causes anxiety and fear of the unknown. It breeds self-doubt, causing us to forget all we've accomplished because we're too busy looking ahead. Those emotions are real and they demand attention. Here are some ways I have found to stabilize them:

Identification

Identifying an emotion and exploring where it's coming from is the first step toward understanding it. For example, I become anxious because I can't control every aspect of my life. I become frantic, grasping at straws attempting to piece together a reason for why things are happening the way they are. The simple act of putting words to these issues has been a good first step to understanding the effect they've been having on my life. Giving a name to whatever it is that's causing us stress allows us to face it more easily, because we can take ownership of the issue, rather than the other way around.

Practice

I have been managing my anxiety, one way or another, for most of my life. I'm learning what works and what doesn't, what's healthy and what's not. We all have our own coping mechanisms to deal with uncomfortable emotions. Some feed them with food while others may mask them with sarcasm. I took to trying to control my anxiety through purging. I felt if I could control what went in and out of my body I could in turn control my life and thus relieve myself from anxiety. I've since recovered from that particular habit, but it's taken time to get to a place where I know how to manage it.

And the process is only beginning, because healthy mechanisms— like yoga, meditation and therapy—only work when we dedicate ourselves to their practice. Through this practice, we can prepare ourselves to react to these emotions in healthier ways.

Awareness

It's important to learn our triggers. They will change over time, but they tend to stay within the same realm. One of my triggers is lack of control. Where others may become anxious when faced with decisions, or having to speak in front of a group, I'm rendered catatonic when I'm not in control of what is happening around me. It does take constant effort to remind myself that I can't control everything, but my effort has begun to prove rewarding. I've learned it's easier to embrace the chaos rather than attempt to control it out of fear. Emotional triggers can be sneaky, so putting the energy into remaining vigilantly aware is the best way to stay ahead of them.

Acceptance

Above all else, accepting the fact that we can't solve all of our problems, and that some problems aren't really problems at all, will bring the most relief. One of the biggest epiphanies I've encountered in this process may be an obvious one, but it wasn't until I articulated it to myself, in my own words, did it truly have meaning: "The future will never exist." That has become my new mantra. Accepting that tomorrow hasn't happened yet, therefore it doesn't exist. It will never exist. It will never be visible or tangible, it is a figment of our imaginations. So it's worthless to pretend we have any control over it. All we have is our present moment, and it is our responsibility to do all we can with it in order to attempt to guarantee ourselves the tomorrow we want.

We all have our own crosses and find different ways to bear them. But in general, we all share one thing: the present. It is something we all share, collectively, and tend to frivolously waste. I encourage us all to attempt to savor it. Life is much more fleeting than we care to admit, which is why we find ways to avoid or escape the present moment. We fear how elusive it is. We hate that it slips through our fingers. But as soon as we embrace it for what it is, a beautiful gift we are all given, we will be able to relish in it rather than run from it. So, be here now.

//

Patience is a practice, not a virtue. A virtue is a behavior showing high moral standards. Patience, the act itself, is virtuous. But more importantly, it is a practice. A practice that takes consistent dedication. Like any habit or behavior, practice makes perfect.

Some days I write a blog post, tackle my to-do list, put on make-up, meal-prep, write another blog post, schedule multiple playdates and declutter the whole house!

Some days I stare at my computer screen, willing it to type words for me.

Every day is different, but what remains the same is my willingness to do the damn thing. Some days are *way* more productive than others, but every day is a step forward. It's all progress.

Don't compare yesterday to today. Don't compare your blog to hers. Don't compare your year one to someone else's year seven.

Be gentle with yourself. Be patient. Take breaks when you need them. Kick ass when you can. You're the only metric determining your success.

Patience involves a lot of waiting. And waiting can be discouraging at times. Waiting can be synonymous with longing, with yearning, with the feeling that something is missing. Waiting is an effect of missing something. And time, it seems, has been convicted as the thief.

My friend gave me a book that asked me to write down four fears and dissect them. I was told to find the root of each fear and see if the four were connected in some way. My four fears were: mortality, settling, imperfection and not knowing. Through my analysis I realized my four fears actually were sewn together with one common thread: time. I was afraid of losing it, wasting it, not having enough of it, not knowing what to do with it.

My biggest realization in this unpacking process was understanding that time is not mine to possess. I don't have time to use it. I live time. I am living in time and space and experiencing it.

It is easy to become possessive of time. As if it is ours alone to take advantage of, to hoard, or to waste. But that just isn't the case. Time doesn't belong to any one of us. So no longer will I complain about not having enough time or wasting my time or biding my time. I will be patient. From now on I will embrace time for what it is: limitless, expansive, universal. And with that much time, patience suddenly becomes an easy practice.

//

I think what it all comes down to is living life on purpose and trusting that we're all in this together. We're all walking the bridge as we're building it.

Collectively, we are all shaped by our own individual experiences. Never forget that just as you have had pieces of your past shape how you think and behave the way you do now, so has that person you're cursing out for not thinking and behaving the way you'd like them to. We all have our own thrilling, complicated, happy, and sometimes painful stories. We must respect that, not judge it.

My humble suggestion? Strive for vulnerability. Take pride in our ability as human beings to be vulnerable, because vulnerability is the ultimate form of strength.

Chapter 16: The Remedy

My husband and I took a trip around the Pacific Northwest one summer. This trip started in Seattle and worked its way down to Portland, through Oregon, down to the country fair in Eugene, and all the way back up again. During our time in Oregon, my husband and I stayed at an intentional community. Some of you might be more familiar with the term "commune." Our friend bought a considerable amount of land with a group of people and they all live on (and off) this land. They've each built their own semi-permanent home, dug an irrigation system by hand from the nearby river to have fresh water and grew a massive garden with all the food you can imagine. They even have toilets that use sawdust to break down waste into compost. They are happy, they are healthy, and, most importantly, they are successfully off the grid.

It is important to note that this is not a new concept. Communities like theirs have been around for quite some time. And not just in our country. For example, in Israel many people live in *kibbutzim*. Each of these communities operate according to guidelines established by their own respective community members. Some all share one bank account, some don't use any money at all. Some communities share all of their resources, some divide responsibilities, some have thousands of people, some have ten.

The community we stayed with had about ten or so people, of all different ages and backgrounds. They each had their own jobs and made their own money. They bought their own food and resources. The one thing they all absolutely shared, though, was their dedication to living intentionally.

This is the one thing I'd say all of these communities have in common: intentional living. Now, what does that mean? In short, it means living on purpose. Being mindful about the choices you're making... for yourself, for your community, for your world. There is a shared mindset within intentional communities, a cohesion that roots them to the same cause. When we stayed with my friend, I learned that this community's unifying thread was a shared love for the land. They owned about forty acres, yet only occupied two. They were preserving the land and letting it remain wild. They thanked the garden for providing fresh food; they thanked the river for offering fresh water. They loved the land and trusted it loved them back.

I get if this isn't exactly your cup of tea. Not everyone can have a relationship with the land quite like this community. But I can bet you understand the idea of caring about something enough to live intentionally and tap deeper into it. Whether it's your love for the land, the sea, animals, your kids, humanity. You get what it means to live with intention. And that's what I want to expand upon. Because most of us aren't living in communes. We don't get to wake up and bathe in a river and grab breakfast from our garden. Most of us wake up in a house, with a kitchen counter full of bills and kids that need to be driven to school and a deadline that needs to be met. But I believe that we can all inject a bit more of intentionality into our daily lives and reap the wonderful benefits of that lifestyle.

I believe one of the best souvenirs to bring back from a trip is a shift in perspective. Below are a few things I brought back from this trip that I try to intentionally incorporate into my daily life in order to feel more connected.

Mindful Eating

As someone who has lived with an eating disorder, I understand what it's like to have a reactive relationship with food. Since I've been in recovery, however, I've learned how to have a more proactive relationship with the food I put in my body. I no longer eat to evade emotions, I eat to thrive. I make choices that fuel my body and help it run at its optimal capacity. I've educated myself on what food is best for me. What I eat has nothing to do with my body image and everything to do with my body's performance. I try to eat my meals sitting down, stopping between bites to actually experience what I'm eating. If I choose to indulge, I do so knowingly. That is to say, I know that brownie isn't going to help my body perform at its optimal capacity...but I also know that **one** brownie isn't going to **keep** my body from performing at its optimal capacity. It's just a matter of being present and conscious about your choices.

Clearing Space

I hate clutter. One, because it's messy. But, more importantly, because it's gluttonous. It shows that I have more than I need. And this is obviously a natural by-product of our consumer-driven lifestyles. Inevitably, we continue to end up with more than we need. So, my method is to stay mindful of that. I consistently clean out my house of clutter or excess. I compartmentalize my home and tackle each space on its own: my closet one week, the kitchen another, the next I'll clean out the office. Some things I will try to sell, other things I happily donate and some just need to get tossed— specifically the mountains of paper that suddenly appear all over the house, like receipts, bills, invoices, and to-do lists. My house is littered with paper, constantly. And no matter how many times I've "opted to go paperless," my physical mailbox is continuously stuffed to the brim with physical paper. So, I am always in the process of collecting and recycling piles of paper from around my house. Decluttering the excess is the best way I've found to clear space in my world. Not only is my physical space clear and functional, but so is my headspace. When everything has a purpose and is in its own place, my head is free to focus on what matters.

Self-Care

This is something I am vigilant about. Mostly, because no one else can do it for me. I can't rely on anyone else to know when I need to rest. Therefore, I am dedicated to listening to my body and knowing when it's nearing burn out. I have put certain systems in place to avoid burnout, such as my meditation and spiritual practice. It is my responsibility alone to know when to speak up and say, "No, not right now, I need a break." That's a trap I'm familiar with, and I don't think I'm alone. We run ourselves ragged to be everything to everyone and expect someone else to say, "You look tired, why don't you take a rest." That is just not how it works. People will take as long as you're giving. And, as the old adage goes, you can't pour from an empty cup. So we must be mindful and tune into our own needs. Know when to stop, lock ourself in the bathroom, and sink into the tub of warm water.

Quality Time

Today, time seems to be our most valuable resource. Mostly because we don't seem to ever have any of it! We are stretching ourselves so thin that there is absolutely no time to just be: to just sit with other humans and connect and engage. That is why we have adapted to this world of screens and messages— it's all surface-level interaction. There is less depth to our relationships because we don't have the **time** to dive deeper. So, I have made it my personal mission to combat that. I am conscious about the time I spend with my friends and family. I make sure it's valuable and connected. I make an effort to unplug and focus all my attention on them. I actively listen to them, I make mindful choices about how we spend our time together. Rather than scream at each other over drinks in some loud bar, we can hang at someone's house and drink wine and catch up. Rather than binge-watch TV shows with my husband for the sake of understanding what everyone else is talking about online, we choose shows that force us to engage in discussion and illicit a response, which leaves us interacting and connecting once the credits roll. I try to host family dinners at the house where we can all sit around the table and, quite literally, break bread. No matter how busy our weeks might have been, we can all sit down at that table for at least an hour and connect.

This practice of incorporating more intention into my daily life eventually spilled over into how I conduct my online life. I now post and scroll with intention.

Have you ever found yourself lost in the scroll?

Have you ever been scrolling so hard on your phone that your hand falls asleep? Or been staring at your phone in bed for so long that your hand gives out and the phone falls on your face? It happens. We are just so in it with this social media machine, to the point where I think a little part of our brain forgets that it's fake... or styled...or paid for.

Life is not all filtered Instagram pictures and styled product imagery and beautiful lattes and handstands on the beach. But some of it is. Some of life is super pretty and fun and positive and worthy of being shared in a four-by-four box, filtered for emphasis.

For better or worse, social media has become ingrained into our existence. It's become natural for us to document and share our lives with the world. But with that comes the flip side, which is the invisible veil that blankets all of that content. The shadow side. The unconscious contract we all sign, agreeing to the filters and the paid posts and hashtags in exchange for a small glimpse at how other people live their lives.

Don't get me wrong: I've ordered the fancy coffee just to take a picture of it. And I've made my husband take pictures of me doing a handstand on the beach. And I'll tell you what— it took about 50 takes before I got even close to it. And even still, I threw a filter on it before posting.

I do less of this now, but I still enjoy documenting my life. I'm not "livin' for the 'gram," but I'll still pose in front of the pretty sunset or dress up in matching outfits with my daughter. Because it's pretty and fun and I want to remember it. I don't post those moments as much because I've started implementing firmer boundaries with how I use social media. But, I'll tell you what: I'm still eating it up when YOU post it.

The gorgeous vacation photos, the month-by-month baby updates, the adorable picture of your dog in his Halloween costume. I live for that shit! And it's okay if you like it, too. I just think we need to start developing a bullshit buzzer in the back of our brains for those moments where we get lost in the scroll and forget those are just tiny, filtered, carefully chosen snapshots of a much larger picture.

//

Self-help has always been a concept I supported, because that's truly what I believe. The only one who can help you is you! Some of us like to victimize ourselves and blame other people for our problems. But the only person who can truly change your life is you. The only way to get the life you want is to go get it yourself. Self-help, help yourself.

So, that's all well and good and I agree with that. But, an entire industry has been built around this "self-help" concept. We've become so miserable and so out of touch with what makes us happy that we are willing to spend billions of dollars for other people to feed us their version of happy. People started to see that other people were willing to pay cash money for this. So, gurus and life coaches and authors and regular people started coming out of the wood-works telling us how to live our best life. They make us believe they have the secret. And they sell it and package it up in all these different and compelling ways, and make a shit ton of money doing it.

And it's not all bad. That much I know. But in the age of the internet, where we are constantly consuming all of the content, all of the time, it's hard to sift through it all. When everybody and their mother is selling their own brand of self-help, it's really difficult to figure out what actually resonates with you. How can we know what our own brand of happy is when we're being sold all of these other people's brands of happy? We don't have time to try all the things and read all the books and buy all the classes and join all the masterminds.

So, what happens? Well, for one, we're left thinking we can't help ourselves. We become overwhelmed. And, eventually, we say *fuck it*. We admit that there's no way we can do all of that. And if we can't do it, we can't be happy. Because there's no way we can go to yoga for 30 days and eat vegan and cut sugar and see a therapist and learn how to manifest with *The Secret* and throw out everything we own and fly to that retreat in the Caribbean and and and and and...

What's worse? All of these methods contradict each other. It's a cavernous spectrum of being told to do nothing and do everything all at once. So we, the masses, the general population, are left feeling lost. We know we don't feel our best. We want to get better. We know we have the power to make ourselves feel better. But we can't grab onto anything and get our heads above water. There are too many life rafts to choose from and it's easier to just float around on our backs, trying not to sink.

We *could* just bunker down and take a long, hard look at our lives and realize what's really making us feel this way. Find the root issue and solve it. But that takes way too much time and energy. We don't have time to stop and reevaluate, recalibrate, reset. We're "too busy."

So, what do we do instead? I'll tell ya! We don't do a damn thing. We continue double-tapping pictures and following other lives that we want ours to look like. We fool ourselves into believing that we're actively bettering ourselves by following these people and liking their posts and buying their books and stacking them up on our nightstands and taking a picture and hash-tagging it and having them re-post it! That's not self-help.

Through social media and this quest for virality and all of that being injected into the self-help industry, the help isn't happening. The work isn't being done. Because it does take a lot of time and patience and effort to put these tools in place and work with them. I've always been a proponent for self-help and figuring out what works for me, sticking with it, falling off the horse and climbing back on again. That's a normal part of life. Things work until they don't. And when they stop working, it's our job to figure out what does.

It wasn't until I fell off the horse especially hard that I had to seriously reevaluate the choices I was making and be like, *some of this shit just ain't workin' for me.* "This shit" being my unhealthy coping mechanisms: self-harm, depression, binge-eating, and social media addiction. So, little by little, I began to cut those unhealthy habits out of my life.

During my many periods offline, I realized that it wasn't social media itself but my relationship with it that was a problem. And since returning, I'm learning how to use the platform to connect with people in a way that works for me and fits my own brand of happy.

A lot of opportunities live online and it'd be silly for me to throw them away because I couldn't figure out how to coexist with the technology. I have to adapt and evolve. We all do, frankly. Because we as human beings weren't built to consume all of this information all at once and to decipher what's worth keeping and what's not. That filter in our brain hasn't developed yet. So I'm trying to build one for myself. And I'm doing that through trial and error.

We don't realize how much white space we have in our lives, white space that we fill up with all of this noise. All of this internet and news and social media and likes and follows and filters. All of the things we are doing all day to stay on brand and to keep our brand going.

And I'm not just saying this to business owners who have online brands. I'm saying this to all of us who are posting to social media with pictures and comments and statuses. We're all keeping to a certain brand that we've created for ourselves. And it takes effort to do that. It's a job. You're a full-time brand manager.

And even still, some of us aren't even posting anything online, but we're still constantly consuming content. My husband, for example, hasn't posted a single thing to social media in years. Certainly not in the six-plus years that I've known him. Yet, he constantly catches himself lost in the scroll, consuming garbage content, slowly slipping into a state of lethargy and self-loathing. Even when we aren't "participating" in the game, we're still playing. We're still mindlessly consuming.

When I eliminated social media from my life, I was able to take a step back and realize how spacious my life really was. I got to witness all of the white space that I'd been filling up with this garbage.

We do have the space to stop and witness our lives. To take breaths and think and unload what's in our head. There *is* that white space working around us. There *is* silence. There *is* stillness. And once the noise of social media is muted, we can use that space to our advantage.

The effort that we put into staying in the know and being the first to know and to always be in-touch and to not miss anything ever is exhausting. I've heard people tell me that's a legitimate fear they have— which freaks me out. After signing off, I had people message me saying things like, "I want to get off social media because it makes me feel horrible, but I'm too afraid of missing something."

People would ask me, "Aren't you afraid of missing something?" And I'd say *NO*. I want to miss things. That's why I signed off. I wanted to miss them. I didn't want them in my face anymore.

The truth is, being off of social media, I did miss out on some things. I wasn't the *first* to know when a big event happened because I wasn't scrolling through Facebook. But I was consuming news in other ways. I'd listen to NPR every day in the car. I'd subscribe to podcasts. I'd follow blogs and consume content that way. I'd read the Skimm'd newsletter to stay up-to-date on current events. I still read about the news and the events and the happiness and the trage-dies. I was still a part of the world. I stayed current. I could hold my own in debates and be informed and educated. And I didn't need Facebook to do that.

I know it's hard to believe, but for a long time people didn't need Facebook to stay in the know or to stay in touch. There were, and still are, other ways to consume news and to stay connected. Social media has just made it stupidly simple and way too convenient. It's like fast food, for your brain. Easy? Yes. Better? Not really.

Right now, the news that we are consuming (especially the way we are consuming it) is so vile. It's toxic. It's not informing us, not keeping us educated. It's dumbing us down, scaring us, keeping us small and trapped. It's not giving us the space to think and extrap-olate and grow and come up with informed opinions and decisions.

Worst of all, we're convincing ourselves that we're not good enough. We're consuming all of this media together and believing we don't measure up to the perfect, varnished lives we're scrolling through.

And that, my friends, is straight-up bullshit.

Being a mom on the internet seems to take the cake when it comes to feeling like a total failure, wouldn't you agree? The unso-licited advice has no bounds.

I get so annoyed when people comment on my parenting. They use the justification that that's how they were raised and they "turned out just fine." My typical response to that unsolicited advice is, "Yeah, but it's been 100 years since then and we've learned a thing or two...so I'm going to go ahead and put on sunscreen and wear my seat belt. K, thanks."

But lately I've been thinking about that very same justification. Being a parent today is like navigating a minefield of guilt. There are so many ways to fuck up and so many people watching and waiting for that fuck-up. The parenting world can unfortunately be super judgmental. And on top of that, we have so many conflicting resources coming out on a constant basis, it's really hard to know if we're doing anything right.

So I got to thinking about how I was raised, because I also seemed to have "turned out just fine." And thinking about all the ways my parents "did it wrong" by today's unreasonable standards really did help me to cut myself some slack. Raising a tiny human is hard enough. But treating it like you're trying to win the parenting Olympics is just stupid. And exhausting. And soul crushing. And unnecessary.

My mom had me via Cesarean at thirty-six-years-old, after a few miscarriages. She quit work to stay home with me. I was formula-fed from day one. She started giving me rice cereal at one month old. I slept on my tummy with bumpers in the crib. I slept in my parents bed well into elementary school. I'd even set up a makeshift bed of blankets and pillows and sleep on the floor next to my mom. I used to watch TV to fall asleep. There was no such thing as organic. No one had ever heard of GMOs. I ate so much sugar—my Cuban grandparents would literally give me a cup of sugar with a spoon to eat. That's a true story. I had a computer in my room. With the internet. Dial-up internet, but still. I'd sleep over my friends' houses all the time. I ate Lunchables every day. I had my birthday parties at Dandy Bear every single year, until I got too old for that. Then I'd have a pool party at my grandparents' house. Every year. The same birthday party. And I loved it. I could count on my hands the number of plane rides I ever took with my parents. I didn't play any sports. Or have any real extracurriculars. I was over-protected and I was overly confident.

And I turned out just fine.

My parents decided for themselves how to raise me. Without the chorus of judgement. Without the encyclopedia of rules. They managed to raise a smart, confident, well-adjusted human being. I may have been raised on cartoons and fake food and teen magazines. But those things don't add up to the amount of love I was raised on and surrounded by. I was encouraged to be happy, to try new things, and to love myself. To have a free spirit and an open mind and a generous heart. So I have a bit of a sweet tooth and some separation anxiety. But all in all, I'd say they did a pretty damn good job.

We've been tricked into feeling this sense of anxiety about our decisions, and it's informing how we choose our paths in life. My generation was raised in the age of the internet, and grew up with everything we ever needed to know right at our fingertips. With so many places to look, it's hard to know which way is right for you. And now, with the advent of social media, we get to watch how everyone else is choosing to do things, and we begin to question our own decisions even further. It's a vicious whirlpool of identity crisis. And we're drowning.

The truth is, it's not about what your parenting or your career or your life looks like to anyone else. Redirect your gaze inward. Look around at your own family. Your own kids. How are they doing? Are they healthy? Thank goodness. Are they happy? Wonderful! I think those are the only two universal standards that everyone should be focused on. The rest is up to you!

I have a few key values I try to focus on with my kids. Along with being happy and healthy, I want them to be grateful, respectful, and curious. From now on, those are the values that will be informing my parenting decisions. Not anxiety. Not comparison. Not judgement. I'm throwing out the last fuck I have to give and I'm refocusing my attention on what I believe matters most: raising good humans.

Chapter 17: Little Voice

This year I got to attend my ten-year high school reunion. It got me thinking about who I was ten years ago and all the things I wish I could say to that girl.

The girl with crazy hair and crazier clothes. The girl who never understood what was cool or trendy. The girl who pretended to be in the marching band because all her friends were in it. The girl who was overly concerned about her grades and her boyfriends and her waistline. The girl with the loud laugh and the crooked teeth. The girl who was sometimes too scared to try new things but somehow always able to speak up for herself. The girl who had no idea what the next ten years were about to bring her, but desperately wanted to.

I'd tell her she doesn't need to go on another crash diet. I'd tell her to buy a hairbrush. I'd tell her not to delete her Myspace and Facebook pages after her boyfriend dumps her because she's going to wish she could see those pictures again. I'd tell her to wear her glasses. I'd tell her to stop sticking her tongue out in pictures. I'd tell her to be nicer to her mom, because she was just trying to protect her from this sometimes scary world. I'd tell her to trust herself. I'd tell her she's still best friends with all the same people. And she still listens to all the same music. I'd tell her she's stubborn but that's what'll get her everywhere she's going. I'd tell her it's okay to not know where she's going.

I'd tell her that's the fun part. I'd tell her she'd never be able to guess where she'd be in ten years. But I'd tell her it's exactly where she's meant to be.

I don't know how it's been ten years since I graduated high school. Sometimes it feels like it was yesterday and sometimes it feels like a lifetime ago. I cringe thinking of the time and energy I wasted worrying about whatever it was I was worrying about when I was a teenager. I look at young girls today and I just want to hug them. I want to scoop them up in my arms and hold them tight. I want them to know how incredible they all are. And beautiful. And worthy. And smart. And talented. I want to tell them everything I refused to hear when I was their age, and I want to tell them until they have no choice but to believe me.

//

As a parent, it's hard not to want to give my kids the world. That's what happens when we have kids, right? We want to give them everything we never had. We want to learn from the mistakes made before us and do better. We want them to have perfect lives. But they can't. Their lives can't be perfect because there's no such thing. Social media temporarily tricks us into believing it is real and it is attainable. But it's not. And we're killing ourselves trying to chase this unrealistic expectation. And while we're busy chasing it, our kids are watching. And learning. And that's not what I want to teach my kids.

I don't want to teach them that they need to be chasing happiness or rushing or busy. I don't want to teach them that they need to be perfect. I want them to know that sometimes life isn't perfect, but that I'll always be there for them when it isn't. And that sometimes, life can be more perfect than we ever imagined. And that I'll be there for those times, too.

So on those days when you're feeling like you're doing everything wrong, just stop for a moment and ask yourself, "Am I loving them?" If the answer is yes, you have nothing to worry about. If you're giving them all the love that your heart can give and then some, you can stop beating yourself up.

It's okay. They'll turn out just fine.

//

Parenting with mental illness has been challenging, but that challenge forced me to develop a new relationship with my anxiety. I'm taking ownership of it. I'm doing my best to stay in front of it and be proactive. I'm not trying to *control* it, because I'm finally realizing that I can't. I can't grip it and tackle it and subdue it. I can't pack it up in a box and ship it off. I can't get rid of it. At least, not as of right now. So for now, I'm accepting it as a part of my life and I'm taking a new, more gentle approach to dealing with it.

I'm learning a lot about my anxiety the more I take time to sit with it. When it comes up, I notice it. I feel it. I don't try to run away from it, because I know I can't. I just let it be there, making me feel all the awful ways it makes me feel. I'm patient with it. Sometimes I'm strong enough to listen to that faint whisper in the back of my head reminding me it'll pass. Sometimes, I'm not. But I do feel a new relationship with my anxiety forming, and I have my self-care tools to thank for that.

I use these tools interchangeably. Some days I manage to touch on every single one. Some days I'm lucky if I'm able to find time to take one nice, deep breath. But I'm learning to not use them as a crutch, as I used to in the past. I'm learning to not depend on routine. I'm learning that change and disorder are major triggers for my anxiety, and thatI lean on routine to feel safe. But that's not sustainable **because routine isn't natural**. Life won't always fall into place exactly as I need it to. So, I'm learning to *go with the flow.*

God, that sounds so cliche. I won't pretend like it's a switch I can flip. But I am learning to pay attention and notice before impulsively and mindlessly reacting. I notice the anxiety I feel when the kitchen is messy or when there are school papers all over the table or when my husband leaves his clothes *next to* the hamper. And instead of rage-cleaning and feverishly organizing, I'm letting myself sit with that emotion. I'm letting myself *feel* the anxiety, knowing what it is and why it's there. And that process has really helped me start to cope with it better.

I'm trying to go with the flow a bit more. I'm leaving the messes. I'm noticing how I feel when I see them. I'm trying to say yes more to situations that make me uncomfortable. I'm trying to laugh more. I'm trying to listen to myself and what I need, and then trying to do more of whatever that is. Some days it's waking up early and exercising. Some days it's going back to bed when the baby takes her morning nap. Some days it's taking a walk. Some days it's writing. Some days I haven't got a clue, so I just sit there and breathe and try to give myself a hug from the inside out. I'm trying to be a better friend to myself.

I'm trying.

That's as much as I can say right now. But I think that's plenty. That's all any of us can do, right? Just try. One step after the other, always keeping your gaze forward. If you're moving forward, you're moving in the right direction.

If this thing doesn't work, then try that thing. If that one doesn't work, try the other. It's all trial and error. And as soon as one thing starts working, something else breaks and you have to try all over again.

That's life. We're in a constant state of trying and learning and growing and transitioning. It never ends. There is no destination. We never get *there*. But we're always **trying** to. And that is a trip worth being on.

Sometimes, that trip can be messy. It can feel like our entire being is an overstuffed suitcase and the zipper just popped and everything flew out all over the room. And we become too lazy or distracted or scared or sad to walk around the room, pick everything up, and put it back together. Because that would mean sorting through what we want to keep and what we shouldn't. That would mean taking the time to face ourselves and work through why we feel this way in the first place. That would mean digging around to try and find the root. And what if we don't find it? What if we're just broken? What if our digging makes a bigger mess, digs a bigger hole, that we can't crawl our way out of?

When I start feeling like this, it is as if my mind, body and soul are three different people. Three different people who are lost and wandering around an abandoned building all searching for the same door. And I know I need to take care of those three people. I need to go find them, grab them each by the hand, and lead them to that door. I spend so much of my life taking care of the people I love. And it is time I start doing the same for myself. Loving my mind. Loving my body. Loving my soul. And showing that love the same way I do for my kids, my husband, my family and my friends. By taking care of them. That is how I must cultivate self-love.

Falling in love is a tricky thing. It takes so much time and then takes no time at all. It's a balancing act of knowing when to be selfish and when to compromise. It's forgiveness and trust and discovery. It's confusing, but exhilarating. Difficult, yet so satisfying. There are many different kinds of love, but the trickiest of them all is the love we must fall in with ourselves.

You see, we can't expect to give ourselves fully to another person, be a strong partner, lead a successful team, or parent our children effectively if we're unsure about ourselves. How can we expect someone else to be happy with us if we aren't happy with us? We all know this to be true, but, man, is it easy to forget. Let us never be too stubborn to deny ourselves the help of these few simple reminders.

1. We don't need someone to love us in order to love ourselves.

I don't understand this notion that pairing up with another person will bring happiness. Isn't it unfair to put that responsibility on someone else? As if once we meet someone, all of the sudden all of our insecurities go away, all of our fears and doubts vanish, that lingering sensation of loneliness and inadequacy just disappears. That's not how it works. We can't depend on someone else to make us whole or happy. We first need to achieve that ourselves, on our own, before we can ever expect to share ourselves with another person. Looking for a partner at a time when we're unhappy being alone is a recipe for disaster. Partners should enhance each other's happiness, not be responsible for it.

2. The self-discovery never ends, we just get better at it.

Sometimes, partners need to pick each other up. Those fears and doubts, they never really go away. We are ever-evolving creatures. And while it is imperative that we discover ourselves and grow individually, we will also continue to grow once we're in a relationship. Different hurdles will spring up in front of us, new emotions will begin to rattle our nerves and shake our security. But it takes being completely comfortable with who we are now, in our moment, to fearlessly look forward to who we will become. The beauty of having a strong partner is that they can offer support in those times when we inevitably begin to question ourselves. But a strong partner must be strong on their own before they can be strong for another.

3. We all get lost. No one gets a map.

Unfortunately, we aren't given a road map to navigate this journey. And as effortlessly beautiful as life can be, it's also rough and dirty and hurts like hell sometimes. We're going to cry gut-wrenching sobs, and question and doubt ourselves, and feel achingly lonely in our own company. But all of that confusion is shaping us. It is helping us find our direction, guiding us down the path to be the people we need to be. The people we can then confidently share with someone else, knowing we don't need fixing and don't need to depend on that other person to show us how to love ourselves.

4. People aren't mirrors, they can't show us who we are.

We can't depend on someone else to show us why we're worthy of unconditional love and affection. We should know. Deep down in our gut, we need to know our worth. That is the only way to trust that we aren't settling for less than we deserve. And to do that, we must look within. Introspection is difficult, and often avoided, but it is so important. Love must first be cultivated within ourselves in order to be given out and then returned. We receive what we put out into the universe. Therefore, we must take the time to nurture and love ourselves, so we can then trust we are receiving only the best love in return. Only what we deserve—no less!

So let us first commit to ourselves before ever committing to someone else. Take the time and put the effort into getting to know ourselves. Test boundaries, try new things, fail, feel rejection, revel in accomplishment. Let us learn what fills us with joy, what gets under our skin, what challenges our ego. We owe it to ourselves and to our future partners. It's not easy, but it is so worth it. Because self-love is the most beautiful thing we can ever give ourselves, our partners, and especially our children.

So go ahead, fall in love.

//

Now, whatever happened to that little girl with the jean short overalls and the butterfly clips in her hair?

Well, she grew up.

She stumbled her way through adolescence and young adulthood, getting bumps and bruises along the way. She fought with her friends over boys, cried over getting bad grades, drank cotton candy-flavored vodka out of plastic water bottles and, on more than one occasion, wore a shirt as a dress.

She worked really hard in school and landed herself what she thought was her dream job. She realized later it wasn't where she was meant to be. She recognized her roots were imaginary, and that she could get up and move and change and try and fail, over and over, until it felt right.

She fell in love with almost everyone she met. She got hurt. She dated recklessly and oftentimes for the wrong reasons. But she met a lot of interesting people with even more interesting stories along the way.

She lost a lot of people she loved.

She grew restless and anxious and desperate to hit fast-forward on her life.

She got smart. She devoured books and learned as much as she could about everything she wanted to know.

She started being honest with herself about what makes her happy and started making more of an effort to seek it out.

She settled down, got married, became a mom.

She wrote a book.

She wrote this book.

That little girl with the unruly bangs and imaginary love affair with Jonathan Taylor Thomas, she wrote this book that you're reading. She's been living inside me all along, waiting to unpack everything I've written here and sift through it with me. Help me find the answers. She is my little voice. And I'm so lucky to have her.

Chapter 18: Closing Arguments

The term *millennial* might conjure up a certain image in your head, and even a certain rage in your heart. You might see little girls and boys winning trophies for losing baseball games. Or teenagers, riddled with entitlement, asking for a promotion at their clerical desk job at your office. Or perhaps you see a whiny, needy twenty-something complaining about their WiFi not connecting fast enough or their bagel having gluten in it.

Yeah, we millennials get a bad rap. We are a generation who is never satisfied. We crave immediacy. We are entitled and selfish and defiant. But, is that such a bad thing? Shouldn't we be? Shouldn't we want to make changes, question the status quo, resist settling? We should be mending the cracks in this system, because clearly no one is doing it for us. And if we don't fix it, we'll just hand it off to the generation that follows, passing the baton of student debt, job dissatisfaction, mental health issues, and addictions off into the hands of our own children.

We're no longer those little kids choreographing dances to Spice Girls songs in our rooms and begging our parents to subscribe to *Nickelodeon Magazine*. We're adults now. We've graduated colleges we were told to attend in order to get jobs we were told would make us money because that would let us buy things we were told would make us happy. And now we're parents, raising children. Raising the next generation. And we're starting to realize we've been fed a bunch of bullshit.

We've been seeing through this bullshit for a while now. Ever since our little fingers have been able to traipse over a keyboard, we've been typing every question that's come to our minds into a search bar looking for answers. But somewhere between asking Jeeves what the meaning of life is and playing M.A.S.H to fantasize about what we'd be when we grew up, we acquired a mountain of debt, found ourselves stuck at a desk, and never really got back around to reading through Jeeves' answers. We followed that dotted line to success, handed down by the generation before us, and ended up at the finish line realizing we're right back where we started. Lost, confused, and full of questions.

And we're so distracted by the noise that's become embedded in the DNA of our generation that we aren't taking the time to sort through and figure out what's real. And I'm afraid if we don't get our shit together now, we'll just continue handing over this broken system to our kids. Generation after generation. Never breaking the cycle.

This is a call to action. Breed the change you wish to see in the world.

We need to lead by example, teaching our children how to exist harmoniously with this technology. They're watching us and learning from us. I urge you to question what you're reading. Set boundaries with social media. Focus on developing meaningful relationships offline. Set out to enjoy visceral experiences out in the world, for the sake of the experience itself, not to post the picture.

My suggestion is to aim to become a more conscious consumer of content. And in order to become more a conscious consumer, we must first learn how to become more conscious in general. And that begins with dropping into our inner selves. Not in a trippy, mushroom-kind of way. But in a more accessible way. Remember who you were as a small child: curious, inquisitive, welcoming. That small child is still there, in each one of us. It's that little voice that's been guiding us all this time, calling to us from the back of our minds and punching us in the gut when something feels off. Whether we've been heeding its intuitive word or not, it has been there. And it's imperative, now more than ever, that we learn how to listen.

When Timothy Leary urged the youth of his time to turn on, tune in, and drop out, a lot of them listened. The hippies of the 1960's began draping themselves in tie-dye, braiding flowers into their hair, experimenting with psychedelics, and opening their eyes to the deeper meaning of life, the deeper connection we all share.

They began understanding that we're all spiritual beings having a human experience, together. That hatch was just beginning to open before a forceful hand came crashing down upon it. The availability of harder, more addictive drugs brought the downfall of a lot of young people. The Vietnam War finally came to an end, causing a lot of the gusto of the movement to dissipate. The pressure to grow up and leave their idealistic optimism behind was too great for some to ignore.

And so the urgency to turn on, tune in and drop out became a faint whisper in the backs of the minds of men and women now shuffling in and out of offices in their suits. They became well-groomed members of a society they knew was inherently flawed. But that knowing, no matter how blatant, never stood a chance against the pressure to fit in. To climb the ladder. To follow.

I don't believe that urgency has ever gone away. I believe now, more than ever, it is imperative that we turn on, tune in, and drop out. However, I'm updating the war cry for the millennial generation just a bit.

I'm urging us to sign off, wake up, and drop in.

CPSIA information can be obtained
at www.ICGtesting.com
Printed in the USA
BVHW030555210521
607794BV00007B/678